YOUR FITTEST FUTURE SELF

YOUR
FITTEST
FUTURE
SELF

**Making Choices Today
for a Happier, Healthier,
Fitter Future You**

Kathleen Trotter

DUNDURN
TORONTO

Cover image: Agnes Kiesz, Pure Studios
Printer: Friesens

Library and Archives Canada Cataloguing in Publication

Trotter, Kathleen, author
Your fittest future self : making choices today for a happier, healthier, fitter future you / Kathleen Trotter.

Includes bibliographical references.
Issued in print and electronic formats.
ISBN 978-1-4597-4128-7 (softcover).--ISBN 978-1-4597-4129-4 (PDF).--
ISBN 978-1-4597-4130-0 (EPUB)

1. Health. 2. Diet. 3. Exercise. 4. Physical fitness. I. Title.

RA781.T76 2019   613.7   C2018-904738-0
                                                       C2018-904739-9

1   2   3   4   5   22   21   20   19   18

 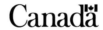 Canada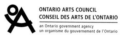

Conseil des Arts du Canada · Canada Council for the Arts · ONTARIO ARTS COUNCIL / CONSEIL DES ARTS DE L'ONTARIO / an Ontario government agency / un organisme du gouvernement de l'Ontario

We acknowledge the support of the **Canada Council for the Arts**, which last year invested $153 million to bring the arts to Canadians throughout the country, and the **Ontario Arts Council** for our publishing program. We also acknowledge the financial support of the **Government of Ontario**, through the **Ontario Book Publishing Tax Credit** and **Ontario Creates**, and the **Government of Canada**.

Nous remercions le **Conseil des arts du Canada** de son soutien. L'an dernier, le Conseil a investi 153 millions de dollars pour mettre de l'art dans la vie des Canadiennes et des Canadiens de tout le pays.

VISIT US AT

dundurn.com | @dundurnpress | dundurnpress | dundurnpress

Dundurn
3 Church Street, Suite 500
Toronto, Ontario, Canada
M5E 1M2

Contents

Introduction

Welcome to *Your Fittest Future Self.* The concept of a fitter future self can feel like a mirage — especially if you have tried many times to adopt a healthier lifestyle to no avail — but creating your unique fitter future you *is* possible.

The two key words are "creating" and "unique." A fitter self doesn't just happen — you can't wish it into existence; it takes work. You have to purposely take the appropriate steps today — because today is the only time we have direct control over what will *create* a different you in the future.

You also have to embrace that you are unique — as we all are. It is unrealistic to think that following any generic program — or even a tailored program that has worked for someone you know and trust — will result in long-term success for *you*. You are the only version of you that exists. Generic programs are just that … generic. Other people's programs are just that … theirs.

Instead of trying to find the perfect diet, workout, and mindset program to follow, *create* something tailored to *you*.

Enter your fittest future self.

Your Fittest Future Self offers you, the reader — the *doer* — a framework built on practical tools that will allow you to parse out the three spheres of health (diet, exercise, mindset) to figure out which of the healthy options will work best for you. You need these tools to curate what I call health *mixes*.

There are three mixes: your NUTRI-TIONmix, your WORKOUTmix, and your MINDSETmix. Together they form your YOUmix. Individualized health mixes are the key to health success. Why? Because we are each unique! There is only one person with your health history, genetics, goals, and life realities: *you*. It is no wonder so many of us continually fall off our health horse. We're trying to use programs created for the masses. We flip from program to program rather than working to understand and learn principles that should underpin our health *process*.

Don't worry. I don't simply explain the tools needed to create these mixes — that would be boring. I offer one-stop shopping and break down the pros and cons of popular diets, workout programs, and mindset philosophies while also empowering you to analyze the information. The result? By the end of *Your Fittest Future Self* you will have both the data and the tools — the cooking classes *and* the ingredients — to create your three unique mixes.

One rewarding outcome of creating these mixes is that it reframes all your past work. Past experiences are no longer something to be frustrated about; rather, they become data — information you can learn from. If you know an element of a diet or a type of workout absolutely didn't work for you, don't add that element to your mix. If you loved a particular element of a diet or a past activity — playing a sport or dancing at clubs — consider joining a team or taking dance classes. Learn from your past experiences so you can create, now, a mix that suits *you* so that you can finally create that fitter you.

Stop trying to find the perfect regimen to follow. Curate a plan that works for you.

As you read the book, remember four things. First, not only will every person's mix differ, but it will also vary and evolve throughout each individual's life. Your mix will not look like your mom's, your favourite celebrity's, or mine, but it will also not look like your future or past mix.

Second, not everything in this book will work for you. Different bits will work for different people, and that's okay.

Third, don't mistake my long-haul approach for an aversion to short-term goals or bursts of intense effort. I love goals. I am constantly setting both long- and short-term goals. Go ahead and have a short-term goal to get in extra great shape for a sporting event or a wedding, but learn to understand these short bursts as part of your long haul, as part of a larger process. Set long-term health intentions that, when appropriate, include short bursts (done in a healthy way) rather than a series of short bursts with no connected thread of intention. More critically, never mistake getting to the end of the burst as an excuse to discard your overall goals and throw yourself off your health horse.

Fourth, the information is structured around the four fitness personalities: gym bunny, competitive athletic gym bunny, time-crunched multi-tasker, and homebody. But that doesn't mean you will find information for only one personality useful. You might find that one personality particularly resonates but that elements of others apply as well.

One of my cardinal rules of life is that you never know what you will learn or what will work, so *be curious*; read everything and see what feels like you. You might be a homebody, but that doesn't mean some of the strategies that work for a gym bunny won't be useful. I'll say it again: *be curious*. Certainty is the opposite of growth. Who knows? Today you might be a homebody, but in the future, you might find yourself able or wanting to go to the gym regularly. A few of the gym bunny lessons might be useful then.

THE MIX CONCEPT

· ·

I have to acknowledge my best friend, Emily, the inspiration behind *Your Fittest Future Self* and the concept of mixes. Emily and I were getting pedicures and discussing diets and fitness routines. I think Emily was asking about the positives of a low-carb diet and what I thought about Lagree Pilates. I was explaining that every health philosophy has pros and cons, that most programs have both useful and bullshit elements, and that finding a sustainable plan is about knowing how to take the good and leave the bad. Emily's response? "You should make this idea of curating an individualized health program the basis of your next book. It is something you stress that is not typical but very helpful." She pointed out that there's no shortage of motivational techniques and diet and exercise regimens, and among so many supposedly healthy options, it is almost impossible to figure out which of the healthy and productive choices are worthwhile. She suggested I write a book that teaches readers how to wade through all the possible choices without becoming overwhelmed, confused, and (worst-case scenario) paralyzed with indecision. So I did!

MY PHILOSOPHY

There are a few key interconnected concepts that underpin the information throughout the book: my fitness and life philosophy is about process, a growth mindset, "working as winning," compassion, joy, owning your choices, and solution-focused thinking. Everything stems from and centres on what I call the Kathleen Cycle.

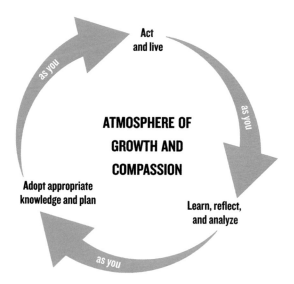

Process

Focus on the health process, not just the end result. Health is a journey with no end date or finish line. Healthy people don't stop being mindful about their health. Sure, you will have small goals along the way — set week- or month-long challenges (I'll be challenging you!) — but realize that the shorter challenges are simply part of a grander long-term process.

The process happens *now* and you have direct control over it. If you want the future you to be different, you have to change your current habits. All you need to do is go as far as you can see … and then you can go further.

Growth Mindset

When you fall off your fitness horse, get back on as soon as possible, and — more critically — get on as a more informed rider. Correct course quickly and learn from everything. Your health process is simply a giant feedback loop. More on that in chapter 2.

Working Is Winning

Part of a growth mindset is embracing that working is winning. The only failure is not trying. If you are working, you can always recalibrate and learn from your experience. If you fall, fall from action not inaction. The only true failure is not trying. We are humans, not robots. Perfection is an unrealistic ask. None of us is perfect — perfection is not possible. Plus, perfect is boring.

Compassion

Do not confuse compassion with letting yourself off the hook or with self-indulgence. Compassion means demanding more of yourself but demanding more because you love and care about yourself, not because you hate yourself. Compassion means caring about yourself (and thus making choices as you would for a loved one), separating your individual acts from you as a person (you ate a cookie — the cookie might not have been an ideal choice, but you are not a bad person), and having a growth mindset (always learning from your experiences). When you cultivate compassion, you form an alliance with yourself — you decide that *you* are your own best friend.

Don't focus on the health mountain — it's too overwhelming! Instead, decide on your first few steps. Once you start, you can tweak your goals and program, but if you never start, you have nothing to build on.

Joy

Joy is key. It is no wonder people find it hard to prioritize motion when motion becomes yet another thing on the to-do list. At the end of a joyless, routine-based day, who would want to work out? To fulfill another obligation, the obligation of training? We want to relax and watch TV; we associate relaxing with throwing off the shackles of adulthood — exercise being one of those shackles.

Goals for Your Fittest Future Self

· · · · · · · · · · ·

1. LEARN — THROUGH FALLING — to make choices your future self will be proud of. If you make a less-than-ideal choice, embrace the learning experience and decide how your future self will react differently.

2. AWARENESS BRINGS CHOICE. Awareness — or consciousness — contains choice. Attention is simply focused consciousness. To make a healthier choice, you first need to be aware of current choices.

3. LIVE LIFE AS IF YOU LOVE YOURSELF; work out and eat well because you love your body, not because you hate it. Love yourself enough to demand more of yourself.

4. BECOME YOUR NON-JUDGMENTAL BEST FRIEND. Stop talking to yourself with contempt and distain.

5. STOP SELF-SABOTAGING BY MAKING FALSE HEALTH CHOICES. Get away from either-or. Work toward this *and* that.

6. EMBRACE THE IMPORTANCE OF CURIOSITY. Certainty is the opposite of growth. Don't live life as if you have everything figured out. Read, be curious, and always be open to change — because after all, where has your current thought process gotten you?

7. LIVE BY THE MANTRA "MY BODY IS NOT A GARBAGE CAN." Act accordingly.

8. **AIM TO EAT FROM THE TOP FEW TIERS** and strive to find as many kiwis as possible. More in chapters 9 and 10.

9. **DEMAND MORE OF YOURSELF** without conflating *more* with body shaming and self-hate.

10. **THRIVE IN YOUR OWN HEALTH LANE.** Figure out what *your* vision of a fit, healthy, happy self is, then work toward that! Work to harness your "you-ness," but the fittest and happiest version of your "ness" you can be; be all-in to health. Lean in!

11. **EMBRACE THAT THE LONGER YOU'VE HELD A HABIT,** the longer it will probably take to replace it with a healthier habit. Give the process time.

12. **CONSIDER MAKING ONE OF YOUR GOALS GREATER INNER STABILITY** — the ability to keep your head and stay on track when given an opportunity to wobble off course. Inner stability includes coping methods, a productive mindset, positive inner dialogue, and self-compassion. The more stable you are on the inside, the more outside forces it will take to throw you off balance and the quicker you will regain balance when it does happen. Negative thoughts, stress, and changing plans are inevitable. Build a stable inner self so you can stay on course.

13. **IMPROVE YOUR ABILITY TO DEAL WITH STRESS.** Think of stress as disproportionate or unproductive attachment — attachment to the meaning we marry to concepts, things, people, jobs, et cetera. A large part of dealing with stress is owning — and letting go of — these meanings. Let go of the meaning you have attached to the perfect body, the perfect exercise week, and even body fat.

The more joy you can find in daily life — I call it finding my pockets of joy — the less of an obligation being healthy is. Plus, the more active activities you find that you like, the happier you will be. It is a positive feed-forward cycle. You feel happier so you move. Moving makes you feel even happier. You start to see joyful activities — going for a walk with your partner, for example — as a privilege, not an obligation, of adulthood. I want you to find the joy in being active.

Owning Your Choices and Being Solution Focused

The only person you can control in this health journey is you; you have direct control over your actions, and on the rare occasions you can't control your actions, you can still always control your reactions. Instead of focusing on the things you can't change and you don't have, focus on what you do have and what you can control. Embrace that daily motion and finding your YOUmix is non-negotiable — and then work at finding the solutions.

WHAT YOU CAN EXPECT IN YOUR FITTEST FUTURE SELF

• •

To make *Your Fittest Future Self* easy to navigate, it includes nine base chapters, a chapter filled with workout plans, an appendix — Kathleen's Recommendations for Growth, Learning, and Joy, which is like an annotated bibliography — and inspirational features, which include my easily recalled mantra-like statements ("Kathleenisms"), challenges, and personal stories.

As you come across a concept or a reference to an author you would like more information on, consult the appendix. Any reference that has really inspired me has been included. Chapter 7 is all about workouts! As you create your WORKOUTmix, refer to this chapter for suggestions and examples. Use the inspirational features as you see fit, but I envision readers rereading a feature or two when extra motivation is required. The first time you read the book, maybe you'll focus on the main text. Then you can leave the book in an accessible location: a coffee table, the office, by your bed. When you want to skip a workout, grab the book and read a few Kathleenisms for inspiration.

Or write some of them on sticky notes and leave them in plain sight for motivation! If you're feeling lost — without a fitness North Star — try a challenge! You'll find these challenges featured in the book — they outline specific ways to galvanize the expansive information (which can feel somewhat nebulous) into distinct challenges (i.e., short-term goals). Short-term goals are a fantastic way to keep you on your horse as you strive for long-term goals. Accomplishing a short-term goal — having a little win — can result in a positive upward health spiral. Feeling alone? Grab the book and read a personal story — learn from my mistakes and growth moments. These stories might be the most important; they will show you that I have been where you are. I'm in this with you!

In chapter 1, Rethinking "Fit," you decide what fit will look like on *you*. People too often fall off the fitness horse because they start with a preconceived, cookie-cutter idea of what a fit person is.

In chapter 2, Getting Out of Your Own Way, I explain that if you want to grow, you have to be willing to let go of the person you have always been. Too often we want to create a different future self while still acting as our current self.

In chapters 3 through 9 we develop your mixes. Chapters 3 and 4 are dedicated to creating your NUTRITIONmix, and chapters 5 and 6 to codifying your WORKOUTmix, with chapter 7 offering workout plans you can put into action. Chapters 8 and 9 focus on your MINDSETmix, a critical component of living your WORKOUTmix and NUTRITIONmix. Action is not the automatic child of education. To live your mixes you need to cultivate a compassionate, tailored, flexible, yet resilient mindset. Mindset is your inner dialogue — your North Star, philosophy, and inner well of resilience and determination. We all have moments of low motivation — I know I do. Instead of being surprised by these moments, and the desires they foster, actively create (then tweak) the mindset to see you through.

In chapter 10, I discuss the interconnectedness of self-trust, compassion, joy, and the ability to respond appropriately. Appropriate responses are productive; they are measured, value-driven, rational, solution-based, and conscious. What needs to overlay every mix — no matter how individualized your NUTRITIONmix, WORKOUTmix, and MINDSETmix are — is an ability to appropriately respond (versus react) to health stimuli. Your ability to respond appropriately is inextricably linked to levels of self-trust.

I BELIEVE IN YOU — YOU *CAN* CREATE THE FITTEST SELF YOU DESIRE

· ·

Adopting a healthier lifestyle can feel overwhelming and demoralizing — yet another obligation — but adopting a healthier lifestyle doesn't have to feel that way. A healthier lifestyle can feel empowering and energizing. Try to think of creating your mixes like going on an adventure or figuring out a puzzle. Have fun learning about yourself and if, at first, the pieces don't fit together, try to figure out why and try again. You *can* do this!

The goal is growth and perseverance! If you are working and learning, you are winning. Stop aiming for perfection. The only true failure is not trying.

Everyone is at a different place on their health journey. Don't unproductively compare yourself to your friend, family member, or celebrities — stay in your own fitness lane! Decide that the only option that is *not* an option is giving up.

As you read, try not to dismiss seemingly obvious advice. Be aware of the dismissive "I know that, so it must not be useful" reaction. As Stephen R. Covey says in *The 7 Habits of Highly Effective People*, "Common sense is not always common practice." You might know the information, but are you embodying it?

My goal is for each reader to learn the tools for their individualized NUTRITIONmix, WORKOUTmix, and MINDSETmix — mixes that both honour your current "you-ness" and life circumstances and help you become the fittest, healthiest, happiest version of you that you want to be. I want you to be able to analyze health information and have the gumption to not be a health sheep and instead say, "Everyone else might think this is the best new regimen, but is it right for me?" I want you to gain the ability to pause before making a health choice and say, "Will this choice make my future self happy? Does this choice align with my personal health value system and the mixes I am trying to create?" I want you to fully lean in to life while fostering a positive relationship with yourself — an alliance with yourself — to become your own best friend. I want you to wake up most days and say, "What will my little wins be today? Where will I find my pockets of joy?"

Drive the bus of your own life instead of letting the bus drive you. Lean in to your health and start working for what you want.

Your fittest future self is waiting — get excited!

CHAPTER I

Rethinking "Fit"

Who exactly is your fitter future self?
What does future you look like?

You have decided you want to create a fitter future self — great! Recognizing a desire for change is the key first step in creating a fitter, healthier future self. The next step is to figure out who exactly your fitter future self will be.

If you are thinking, I want to look and be fit. Fit is fit. What is Kathleen talking about? Don't worry. That is a common response. Fit is a word often thrown around as if there is one monolithic version of fit — as if fit will look the same on everyone. Fit not only looks different on everyone but will also look different on the same person as they age or as their life realities change. Take my dad: he used to

play hockey and only hockey. Now that he is seventy, he plays fewer games per week so he can have time to strength train, garden, bike, and do some Pilates with me. He views these new additions as activities that will keep him mobile enough to play hockey for life. In my twenties I completed a full Ironman, eight half Ironmans, and ten marathons. I thrived on endurance events. Now I gravitate toward shorter runs and Pilates. Why the change? Possibly because I no longer feel the need to prove myself, and possibly because I am concentrating more on my work. Either way, my vision of who I want Kathleen to be — the way I want to spend my time and what I value — has changed. Maybe next year I will do CrossFit. Who knows? The immense possibilities life offers are among the incredible privileges of being alive.

The problem with the current widespread, immutable, one-size-fits-all interpretation of *fitness* and *fit* is that it is, at best, unrealistic and, at worst, highly unmotivating.

You might be wondering why this chapter isn't called Rethinking Health. I purposely use *fit* rather than a broader term such as *health* for two interconnected reasons. First — and most important — the title of the book is *Your* Fittest *Future Self.* To create that fittest future you, you have to first understand how fit will look on you: What is your understanding of fit? How will you embody your understanding of the word? Who is this future you? Second, the title of my first book is *Finding Your Fit.* Why is this pertinent? For me, *fit* is a loaded word. Your fit is not just your jean size or how many push-ups you can do. Your fit is the interconnection between

Value Alignment

• • • • • • • • • • •

Notice my emphasis on what I value. I will circle back on values and value alignment throughout *Your Fittest Future Self.* You need to clarify who you want to be and how you want to act. Align your future self's *intended values* with the values you are willing to live today! Then, take each health decision as a sliding door moment — a chance to act in alignment with (or in opposition to) your value system. Before you make a health choice, pause to decide if the act is worth it; ask yourself, Does this choice align with the value of who I want to be? Remind yourself that regardless of your aspirational values, in the end, for your health, the actions you live matter more than the actions you think about living. Or to quote Stephen R. Covey, "Life is a product of your values not your feelings," and "Life is a product of your decisions not your conditions." So, figure out your values and make the appropriate decisions.

the activities that work best for your body, your relationship to your body, your inner sense of worth, your history, your goals, and how your understanding of health and wellness plays out — how it *fits* — on your body.

People too often fall off the fitness horse because they let preconceived ideas of what a fit person is inform their image of health success. A stereotypically fit person drinks protein shakes, has washboard abs, and trains daily. The problem is, why even start working out when the image of what you are trying to become seems so unachievable? This unattainable version of fit becomes yet another way we self-sabotage, indulge in false either-or choices, and let ourselves off the hook. In short, we don't change or evolve, and we spiral further down the rabbit hole of "I always fail whenever I try. I am doomed to be unhealthy. Why even try?"

WHAT'S YOUR FIT?

· ·

Before you read the remainder of the book to learn strategies that will help you form your fittest future self, it's important to figure out what *fit* means to you. What will fit look like on you? Here are some questions to think about.

➡ How old are you?

➡ What are your genetics?

➡ What are your financial realities?

➡ What are your past injuries?

➡ How much time do you realistically have to commit to movement?

➡ What is your exercise personality?

➡ Do you need to work out at home?

➡ Do you thrive on competition?

➡ Do you like group exercise classes?

➡ Are you so busy you have to fit motion into your daily life?

The Four Fitness Personalities

· · · · · · · · · · ·

The **HOMEBODY** mainly trains at home, whether for comfort, cost, or convenience.

The **GYM BUNNY** mainly trains at the gym or does group exercise classes.

The **TIME-CRUNCHED MULTI-TASKER** finds ways to pepper movement into their daily life: they take the stairs, walk their dog, and possibly commute to work on their bike.

The **COMPETITIVE ATHLETIC GYM BUNNY** thrives on competition and loves team sports or fitness classes like CrossFit.

Of course, there are crossovers, and the categories are malleable and will (and should) change as your life realities change. For example, during busy times at work you might have to be a time-crunched multi-tasker when ideally you would be a gym bunny. Or maybe in-season you primarily play a particular sport and thus are a competitive athletic gym bunny, but in the off season you prioritize strength training and are a gym bunny. Do you. Be you. *Do* and *be* are active words. Pick the personality combinations that are realistic and that work for you and get moving — get *doing*. Act. Embrace the mindset that fitness is a daily non-negotiable, and then figure out which personality will make that daily motion happen.

WHAT IS HEALTHY?

· ·

What does fit and healthy mean to you? Too often, two options — two extremes — exist. Either a person is dedicated, absolutely on their program, and trying to look like a movie star or in the zone of self-acceptance. Typically, neither extreme is productive. Looking like a movie star is — for most people — not an attainable, realistic, or healthy goal. Creating a movie star aesthetic demands intense dedication layered onto all-star genetics — a laser focus on diet and exercise that most of us are not willing to have. That degree of dedication often ends up bordering on unhealthy compulsion.

On the other end of the extreme lies the idea that being healthy is about absolute self-acceptance devoid of a need for growth. While I absolutely advocate self-love and compassion, being healthy does not mean adopting the attitude that you love yourself enough to accept your-(unhealthy)-self just the way you are. Too often the "I love myself enough" attitude is used to justify self-indulgent, unhealthy behaviours by couching them in the legitimate psychological end goal of self-love. The thing is, when you actually love yourself, you want to make healthy choices, not excuse unhealthy behaviours and thoughts.

Wanting to look like a movie star and staying stuck out of a pretense of self-acceptance are two of the most prevalent philosophies of health and together are an example of a false choice. When I suggest figuring out what health looks like for you, I don't mean simply finding the balance between those two points. *Balance* implies that to be healthy you have to find a perfect middle ground. What I want you to decide is what works for *you*. To most, my version of health normal — my ideal balance — would feel extreme. That is okay. It works for me.

Instead of looking for the middle of two socially constructed polar opposites — or even caring about any socially constructed concepts of health — find the version of health that works for you, one that includes a WORKOUTmix, NUTRITIONmix, and MINDSETmix that are both individualized and open-ended. Health has no end date.

Creating an individualized MINDSETmix is not an "if you have time" aspect

False Choices

· · · · · · · · · ·

What is a false choice? A false choice is an either-or choice that we set up — a version of brain propaganda — that allows us to justify unhealthy behaviour. For example:

- Either I go to the gym for an hour or I skip my workout entirely.
- Either I eat well today or I eat badly.
- Either I do my run or I snooze my alarm too many times to do the full run so I might as well keep sleeping.

Can't spend an hour at the gym? Go for thirty minutes and do intervals. Or work out at home. Have an unhealthy work dinner booked? Make the best choice possible and eat well the rest of the day. One treat is not the same as ten treats. Snooze your alarm? No problem: do a shorter interval-based run. Don't self-sabotage. Some movement is always better than none. False choices are simply a flavour of self-sabotage, a concept I will discuss in detail in chapter 9.

of adopting a healthy lifestyle. The right mindset is critical; your mindset overlays every health choice you make. Your mindset — your inner dialogue — allows you to dispute your negative brain propaganda and form appropriate responses. Once you have a strong mindset, the ability to act will follow.

Ditch the body shame. Strive to honour who you are now — your you-ness — while understanding who you want to be, all within an atmosphere of compassion and growth.

Striving for the "perfect" body is just another way to hustle for approval from others and from yourself. The perfect body doesn't exist. Perfection is not possible; no one I have ever met who has what others would deem the perfect body thinks that their body is perfect. We all are our own worst enemies and critics.

I don't want to turn you into a whole new you. A *new you* implies that there is something wrong with the original version. Instead, I want you to learn to love and value yourself. I want you to be the great person you are, just a more active and health-conscious version. I want you to be the fittest future you that you envision!

A sad truth about my relationship with my body is that I didn't even own a bikini before I was 32. I was too uncomfortable in my own skin. Then at 32 I woke up and thought, What am I waiting for? Today is the day to be proud of who I am. Being proud of me and existing in an atmosphere of growth and compassion are not mutually exclusive. I think I always thought that as long as I was still working on me, I couldn't be proud. Wrong. In fact, the prouder I am and the more compassion I have for myself, the easier it is for me to grow and learn. I know now that I can want to improve my strength or running speed while still loving myself and my body enough to be seen in a bikini. I don't have to wait until I have accomplished all of my growth to love myself. As you strive toward your fittest future self, do so while fostering an inner sense of worthiness. I know that this is easier said than done. But the more worthy you feel, the easier it will be for you to adopt and maintain healthier habits.

Genetics

· · · · · · · · · · ·

When deciding on your goals, make sure to respect your genetics. Genetics predispose you to react to food, exercise, and your environment in certain ways, but they're not an excuse for unhealthy behaviour. Genetics are simply one more reason to set realistic individualized goals. Embrace who you are! Don't expect exercise to make you someone you are not. As I often tell myself, unrealistic expectations are the seeds of discontent. Realistic expectations are the seeds of contentment.

Instead of wasting energy unproductively comparing yourself to your friend, a celebrity, or even your mother, use your time effectively and become the fittest, most aware, and happiest version of you that you can be. Set realistic goals that are based on your body, and remember: moving is always healthy, regardless of how it makes your body look. Establish multiple goals that make sense for you and set yourself up for success! As my dad says, "Take your genetics and hit a home run."

STRATEGIES FOR RETHINKING FIT

· ·

So, how do you rethink fit? Here are some strategies.

ALIGN YOUR GOALS WITH YOUR IDENTITY AND VALUES. Embrace both the final result you desire and the effort it will take to reach that result. The amount of work you are willing to actually put in to reach your goal — versus what you wish you would do — has to align with your values and your goals.

To successfully achieve any goal, you can't just be okay with the intended result (for example, losing twenty pounds); you have to be okay with the process (the work that goes into dropping the weight). Be realistic about the work you are willing to do. If the work needed doesn't align with your values and willingness to persist, you will not continue. For example, working out after work might seem ideal for your waistline, but if you value family dinners more than your waistline, you will eventually stop going. Find a realistic solution: perhaps involve your family in the cooking, alternate nights of family dinners with gym workouts, shorten your workouts, work out at home or in the morning, or shorten family dinnertime.

Another example is the way I negotiate social situations. I have clients who feel compelled to eat food when they are at someone else's house. To use Gretchen Rubin's paradigm from *The Four Tendencies*, they are "obligers." To use Kathleen-speak,

> There is a difference between aspirational health values (your health wishes) and practised daily values. You can't do what you have always done and expect your future self to be different. Either decide you are okay with your current values, habits, and identity, or match your goals to what you are willing to do.

Every choice in life — including one you make to reach any goal — has a cost; to repeatedly make any choice, you have to be okay with the cost. All choices have consequences. Decide which consequences you can live with, and which ones you can't.

their value system says that passing on the host's food is rude, and being polite is more important than sticking to their nutrition rules. For them, abstinence at a party is unrealistic — the cost of saying no to a friend is too high. They pay their cost with their health. For me, my health is paramount; I say no to food all the time. I am more than okay with saying, "no, thank you," politely, but firmly. Or I offer to bring a healthy option so I have something to eat. I have decided that the cost of this choice — some people don't love when I say no — is almost always worth it. I know my friends know me, so I am confident they don't believe I am acting out of malice or cruelty. My future self is happy with the choice. Every choice has a cost. Decide what cost you are willing to pay.

Goal Support

· · · · · · · · · · ·

I suggest talking about your goals with others. Stating something out loud can help to solidify its realness, and the more people who know your goals, the more accountable you may feel. And, as Tim Ferriss talks about in his podcast, *The Tim Ferriss Show*, others have the objectivity to notice changes in our overall "way of being" that we are too close to see. This is significant because when you want to quit because nothing has happened, your best friend might be able to inspire you to stay on your path with comments like, "Since you have been eating better you are consistently in a better mood," or "Since you have been exercising you don't seem to be in pain after we go walking."

Your goals have to connect to what you can actually live with and to your identity. Changing a health habit is going to be almost impossible long term if it conflicts with your identity. My identity is very much tied to being a health professional, which is part of why I can say no to unhealthy food.

I also have clients who are within their healthy weight range but who want to lose a few pounds for aesthetic reasons. The closer they are to the low end of a healthy weight range, the harder it will be for them to lose weight — it takes proportionally more work. Many people say they want to lose five pounds, but when it comes down to the

identity shift and values that it would take to reach that goal (for example, no alcohol and virtually no sugar), they decide that in the end it is not worth it.

Einstein reportedly said, "Insanity is doing the same thing over and over again and expecting different results," as well as, "If you want different results, you have to try different approaches." Learn from your old ways of being but know that you have to act differently now if you want your future self to have different habits, values, and identity markers. At every moment decide to either engage with the choice that will produce your fitter future self or engage with your old identity. Align what you are willing to do with who you want to become.

STOP THE SHAME CYCLE. Putting yourself a shame spiral (e.g., I ate this cookie, so I am worthless and thus might as well eat another one) is not compassionate or productive. Learn to note the problem, learn from it, and move on.

In previous works, I have written that "guilt is counterproductive." I want to amend that slightly. *Shame* is counterproductive and emotionally and physically damaging, but guilt can sometimes spur some people into action. By *guilt* I mean the feeling of regretting a specific action, as in saying to yourself, I wish I had not eaten that cookie. Shame, on the other hand, is conflating making a less-than-ideal choice with being a bad person. When you fall into the shame cycle, you get into a trap of thinking, *I did X; therefore, I am worthless.* Feelings of worthlessness do not breed self-efficacy, positive feelings, or productive action.

I am not motivated by guilt. I am motivated by the fact that I know being active will make my future self feel better, more energized, and empowered. But if feeling guilty spurs you to action, use it; if you can learn from the guilt and make better choices next time, great. Just don't let guilt melt into shame. Shame is not helpful for anyone.

How do we break the shame cycle? The three tools that help me break the shame cycle are choosing language carefully; journaling experiences, which includes keeping an inventory of successes; and always having a growth mindset. In *The Gifts of Imperfection, Daring Greatly, Braving the Wilderness,* and *Rising Strong,* Brené Brown highlights the importance of "speaking your shame." Why? Because in her language, silence breeds shame; when you don't "speak" a shame story, the unresolved feelings of shame will fester and shape everything you do — all choices, including food choices. So find a way to articulate your shame story in an arena where you will not be shamed further. For me that is talking to my therapist; my partner, James; or my mom. Find your person, or journal and write your story to yourself. Get it out in a non-judgmental context. Speak it so it does not own you. Or to use meditation discourse, "name it to tame it."

I. CHOOSE YOUR LANGUAGE CARE-FULLY. First, stop using language that undermines your self-efficacy. Own your experiences. Instead of saying, "I couldn't work out today," say, "I decided to prioritize something else." Instead of "I have to exercise," say, "I want to work to improve my X." Instead of "My husband cut up brownies so I had to eat them," say, "My husband went to the trouble of making brownies, so I decided that having a small amount was worth it." Second, stop with the belittling and degrading self-talk. Talk to yourself as if you like yourself, as you would talk to your child or someone you love. Don't let yourself off the hook, but remind yourself that you are human.

2. **INVENTORY YOUR SUCCESSES.** Each night take the time to inventory your successes. When possible, actually write down two or three things you did well. Celebrate little wins.

Preparation.
Preparation.
Preparation.
Schedule —
if it is not
in the schedule
it won't happen.

Don't just note the wins, though; take stock of the strategies you used to accomplish the wins so you can reproduce them.

3. **HAVE A GROWTH MINDSET.** A growth mindset is the ability to non-judgmentally learn from every experience. Instead of berating yourself over a regrettable choice, note what you learned from the experience. Did you overeat at a party because you felt out of place? Because you stood next to the food table? Because you were too tired? Then learn from these experiences. Get back on your health horse as a more informed rider. We will circle back on this concept throughout *Your Fittest Future Self* — harnessing this ability is paramount.

4. **LEARN TO PARENT YOURSELF.** Schedule your life as you would your child's. Apply the same amount of mindfulness to your own nutrition as you would for a loved one. Talk to yourself in a way you would want your child or best friend to talk about themselves.

After fifteen years as a trainer, I have noticed a distinct pattern. Too often there is a disconnect between what clients think is good enough for their loved ones and what is good enough for them personally. Too many people (especially mothers) can outline in detail the healthy choices they make for others but find it nearly impossible to implement the same choices for themselves.

We all know (for the most part) what is healthy. Fries or a salad? Vegetables and hummus or a chocolate bar? Water or coffee? The answers are often obvious — most healthy choices are not complicated. The problem is, when it comes to our own health, knowing and doing — especially doing over the long term — are two very different things.

The key phrase is *our own health*. Most of us prioritize healthy choices for others (like a child or an elderly loved one), yet we find ways of letting ourselves off the hook. You know what I mean: "I can eat that just this once" turns into eating it for weeks; "I will work out Monday" turns into three Mondays from now; "I can watch another hour of TV instead of sleeping since it is a special occasion" leads to the de-prioritizing of sleep becoming a habit.

Love yourself. Period.

I have learned to ask my clients to consciously make choices as if they were making them for someone else. Regarding exercise, that means *actively s*cheduling your life as you would your child's life. Most people I meet actively plan their children's activity schedule; they know that if they don't schedule in movement, their kids will sit and play video games or do something equally inactive. Unfortunately, they often don't actively schedule and prioritize their own exercise regimen. The key word is *actively*. Actively schedule your activity as you would your child's.

Regarding nutrition, *apply* the same amount of mindfulness to your own nutrition as you would for a loved one. You wouldn't expect your kids to eat food off your plate, snack before dinner, or mindlessly grab a chocolate bar at three o'clock, but that is how most parents I work with feed themselves.

For general health, *establish routines for yourself as you would for your family.* For example, create sleep, morning, and bedtime routines. Most parents I know establish (or aim to establish) fairly distinct — particularly morning and bedtime — routines for their children; routines and habits simplify family life by setting expectations and diminishing cognitive thought calories. Do the same for yourself. Create predictable health algorithms (routines) that will serve you: set your workout clothes out the night before, do a predetermined number of push-ups and squats as soon as you get out of bed, or place a glass of water on your nightstand that you drink before your feet hit the floor. Spare your cognitive burden so you can apply your energy to your unique strengths. Stop wasting your energy asking yourself, Will I or won't I do X healthy habit today?

Last, talk to yourself in a way you would want your child or best friend to talk about themselves. Get rid of your destructive internal dialogue. You wouldn't let your best friend or child talk badly about their body and self-worth; why is it okay for you to berate yourself? Obviously, be honest. Don't tell yourself you are making healthy choices if you're not. But don't metaphorically flog yourself with unproductive self-hate.

Work to form an internal dialogue that you would be proud of your child, best friend, spouse, parent, or in my case, client, for having. Foster an alliance with

yourself. Become your own compassionate best friend.

Become mindful of your exercise and sleep habits, your nutritional choices, your internal self-talk, and even the people you surround yourself with. You wouldn't want a loved one swindled by an amoral "friend" — pick your own confidants just as diligently. Love yourself; don't let people walk all over you.

If you're not a parent and don't have an elderly dependent, and the idea of living how you would want your child or parent to live is not helpful, find another way to apply this concept. We all have people we care about; aim to apply the same standards to self-care as you apply when caring for your loved ones.

 For the next month I dare you to make all of your health choices as if you were making them for someone you care deeply for — an elderly parent, your child, or someone else who is important to you. In my case, I don't have a child, so I often ask myself, What would I tell my client to do?

REFRAMING SHOULD

In general, I am not a fan of the shoulds in life. I'm not suggesting you stop doing things you don't want to do. But it's important that you own your actions because you choose to do them, not because someone says you should. For example, forcing yourself to work out and eat healthy food because you think you should typically leaves you feeling deprived. Who wants to make healthy choices when it feels imposed? Instead of saying something like, "My doctor says I should eat more vegetables and less sugar," say, "My doctor recommends more vegetables and less sugar. I read the relevant literature and she's right. I'm going to eat more vegetables because it will make me feel better, and in the long term it will reduce my risk of multiple disorders and diseases." This might sound like semantics, but it's not. In one version, you are thinking of doing something because you have been told to. But unless you can find a way to internalize the choice — to create self-efficacy — the choice will only last for so long.

PERSONALIZE YOUR FIT

The key to finding your fitter future self is learning how to make choices that *fit you*, without grounding your choices in someone else's concept of what a fit or healthy person should look like. I want you to be able to personalize what healthy and fit means for *you*. Let go of what other people think. Do what is best for your future self — do you.

While doing you, strive for appropriate responses rather than knee-jerk emotional reactions. Don't belittle your feelings. If you feel guilty or frustrated, own that — but don't fan thoughts into a full-on shame assault. Toxic brain propaganda is not productive, and listening to toxic brain propaganda will not help you become the future self that you want to be. When it comes to health, the complex paradox is that you have to learn how to honour your you-ness and your emotions while not letting your thoughts become

> You are enough. You are worthy. Your health is important, so prioritize daily movement and the consumption of nutritious food. Your body is not a garbage can — don't put garbage food into it.

such a big deal that they derail your progress. Appropriate responses — rational, measured, and productive responses — will be discussed in detail in chapter 10. Until then, know that one main trick to appropriate responses is embracing the power of the pause. When you find yourself shame spiralling, setting unrealistic fitness wishes rather than goals, or deviating from your health plan, make yourself pause. Pausing will help you stop simply reacting. Disconnecting from the immediacy of a moment is the key to not giving in to brain propaganda such as thinking you want that second piece of cake. More on negative brain propaganda in chapter 3.

Become more mindful of your health choices, but don't wish to be a new you in the process. Instead, work at becoming a version of you who loves yourself enough and has enough self-compassion to exercise and eat well. Create a few helpful internal hashtags or mantras. I find #IAmWorthyOfSelfCare and #WhatWouldMyFutureSelfWantMeToDo? very helpful — they both remind me that my health quest is something I am doing for myself.

Eating fresh berries is a present to yourself, not a punishment. Deciding to eat processed crap full of preservatives is not a prize. If you always put others first, remember that you deserve the same care that they do. Try to give yourself the same attention and time you give to others. Take the skills currently reserved for your friends and family and devote them to your health!

Decide what your image of a fit, healthy, and happy you will look like — the values and habits you want your future self to have. Now, make it happen.

CHAPTER 2

Getting Out of Your Own Way

Change your actions — create a fitter future self — by questioning your current assumptions, mindset, and habits; strive to exist in an atmosphere of growth and curiosity.

Certainty is the opposite of growth. I am assuming, since you are reading this book, that you want to grow and evolve. If so, let go of — de-attach from — what you always do. The spelling *de-attach* is intentional. I am trying to emphasize the space you need to create from whatever you are attached to. Figure out why you are attached to a particular thought, action, or feeling, and literally separate your body and mind from that unproductive attachment. Question what you consider to be common sense assumptions and actions; doing what you always do and believing what you have always believed will create a future self who is a slightly older copy of your current self. Change your actions by questioning your current assumptions, mindset, and habits; exist in an atmosphere of growth and curiosity. Certainty only leads to more of the same. A surefire way to stay stuck as the current you — with your current health — is to be certain of everything you know and to stay married to your current values, assumptions, and daily habits.

This chapter is critical before mix making. The work outlined here has to be done before you can create any of your mixes. Curating any mix revolves around picking strategies that will work for you. Before you can know what will work for you, you have to be aware of your current thought patterns and loops, have perspective, be ready for growth, and be open to change. The information in this chapter sets you up for success, not just in the MINDSETmix chapters, but when curating all your mixes. The information in this chapter will allow you to go into the experience of curating your mixes with enough personal knowledge and perspective to do it appropriately. Without an awareness of your current habits and an openness to change, you will simply, consciously or unconsciously, create a mix based on old versions of you, based on old assumptions — those mixes will simply create another copy of your current you.

I ended chapter 1 advising you to make your future self happen — to decide what your image of a fit, healthy, and happy you will look like and then actively work toward that image.

I am sure you are thinking, *Kathleen, if I knew how to make my health happen,* *I would have done it already.* I get it. Making something happen is easier said than done!

A large part of making a health change happen is informing yourself about relevant health information and learning how to parse out the recommendations that are appropriate for you — that way you know what changes are even worth the effort. It is extremely frustrating — not to mention demoralizing — to make multiple health changes but see no results. The key is to learn which habits will, for you, elicit the most change; find the 20 percent work that will elicit 80 percent change. Too many of us attempt to change life habits that won't have strong enough positive feedback. Linchpin habits — sometimes called cornerstone habits — will differ from person to person. I will explain the process of figuring out which health recommendations will give you the most bang for your habit buck in chapters 3 through 9.

Now — and this is key — knowledge is only part of the puzzle, and often it is the least important piece.

Dr. Fordyce, a seminal thinker in cognitive behavioural theory, pain management, and movement re-education is widely attributed with saying some iteration of, "Education is to behaviour change as spaghetti is to brick." Having one doesn't change the other.

We all know the benefits of working out and eating well, but when it comes to our health, knowing and doing — especially doing over the long term — are two very different things. Stephen R. Covey reiterates this point in *The 7 Habits of Highly Effective People* by positing that creating a habit or mindset change requires the intersection of knowledge, skill (practical how-to skills), and desire (motivation). Knowledge is not enough. (Luckily for you, all three components, not just the knowledge piece, are outlined in this book! If I could include a wink emoji here and still respect myself as a writer, I would.)

You can research and understand the benefits of making a health change, and you can figure out which habit changes will make the biggest difference for you, but until you are ready to change, until you decide to change your mindset around health, logical information just won't stick. Health is a process, and in order for long-term changes to occur, you must want — and be ready — to be part of the process.

Two elements will make actively being part of your health process possible.

➡ **First, you have to learn how to — productively — stay in your own lane.**

➡ **Second, you have to embrace the importance of growth and curiosity.**

Don't get frustrated by the process! W Timothy Gallwey offers a useful metaphor in his book *The Inner Game of Tennis*: Think of your habits like grooves in a record. Every time you act, you create a slight impression on the record. The more often you do the same action, the larger the groove becomes — the needle of the behaviour goes deeper. Deeper grooves usually require stronger and smarter strategies for successful change — and a higher level of compassion and desire for growth. The longer you have had a particular health habit, the deeper your groove will be. The deeper the groove, the harder the work, and the longer the journey out. Keep trending positive. Forward is the only direction that offers the potential for new and improved health habits.

THRIVE IN YOUR OWN LANE — DO YOU

"Stay in your own lane" has long been a go-to Kathleenism, although recently, I tweaked it slightly. Why? It is too often misunderstood as an instruction to ignore others, never be competitive, stop growing — basically resign yourself to being who you are and do whatever you want. This interpretation is the opposite of what I intended. So, now I use a new iteration: "Thrive in your lane."

Don't simply exist or survive in your lane. Instead of being resigned to being who you are and thus being stuck, be proud of what you were born with and your experiences thus far; use your genetics and experiences as a jumping off place to understand what your model can do. As Angela Duckworth states in her book *Grit*, not everyone can be an Olympic athlete, but with grit (perseverance and pluck) almost all of us can function at a higher level — a level closer to our genetic ceiling. Too many of exist at the low end of our genetic window. Be proud of your lane. Use your lane to help you become the best version of you that you can be.

Alternatively, while in your lane, note what others are doing and respond in a way that both honours who you are and serves your future fitter and happier self. Don't conflate other people's needs, goals, and position on the highway of life with your needs, goals, and position. Note their actions (Are they staying in their own health lane? Reacting with ego? Acting out of insecurity?) and then react appropriately with a reflective, mature, positive response. Strive for healthy competition; compete in a productive way, not in an ego- and judgment-filled, perfection-driven way. Doing you in your lane might be competitive — maybe you enroll in a healthy fitness competition at work or train to win a race. Think of healthy competition as analogous to healthy striving instead of perfectionism. Aiming for perfection sets you up for failure. It is an impossible goal and the need is driven by insecurity and unworthiness. Healthy striving is the positive way to work toward the most perfect version of you possible. Staying in your own lane involves healthy

> Aiming for perfection sets you up for failure. Healthy striving is the positive way to work toward the most perfect version of you possible.

competition that is not emotionally reactive and reflection and personal growth.

Everybody is scared and broken. You are intimately familiar with your scared and broken bits — your metaphorical (and sometimes literal) warts — but you are primarily only privy to other people's manicured lives and, typically, makeup-covered faces. It is easy to create an internal narrative — especially when we voyeuristically watch people on social media — that others are happy, have fantastic relationships with their friends and family, are always energetic and happy, and have life figured out. They don't. Since my life is so public — I post all of my health and workout antics on Instagram stories — I relearn this lesson almost daily. People think "you are always so energetic" or "you have such a great relationship with your mom," with the implicit complaint that they don't have what I have. I remind them that my life on social media is curated, as everyone's is. Just picking what you post is a curation process. To offer perspective I will share scenarios when I was tired, or instances when friends or family had a squabble directly after a happy loving interaction on social media. I did not post the disagreement. These ebbs and flows of life simply make me human. Even people who seem to have it all figured out don't. Have compassion for yourself and others, and stay — and thrive! — in your own lane. It is unproductive not to.

STRIVE TO EXIST WITHIN AN ATMOSPHERE OF GROWTH, CURIOSITY, AND ACTION

· · · · · · · · · · · · · · · · · ·

What makes or breaks an individual's health process is the willingness to embrace the mindset that to create a fitter future self, you have to exist within an atmosphere of growth, curiosity, and *action*.

I am sure the advice that to change you have to be willing to learn and grow

> You can't just know what is right — you have to act on it. Embrace the notion that to get different results — a fitter future self — you can't continue to repeat the same thoughts and actions.

Certainty is the opposite of growth. Don't let your love of being certain and right stop you from moving forward. If you want to grow you have to be curious. If you want to stay stuck — locked forever as the same person you have always been — go ahead and be certain about everything you know and stay married to your current daily habits.

sounds obvious, but in my experience it is the biggest missing link for most of us. Most of us want to be able to create a different future self while still acting as our current self.

To evolve and produce your fittest future self — yes, you produce the person you want to be — your thought process has to be malleable and flexible. Embrace what Carol Dweck refers to in her book *Mindset* as a "growth mindset." You need to question your current thoughts and assumptions, and when you fall off your fitness horse, make sure you lean in to that fall; instead of being discouraged, be intrigued and curious. Ask *why* you fell. That way you can make a more informed decision next time.

Aim to exist within an atmosphere of growth, curiosity, and action.

WHAT DOES AN ATMOSPHERE OF GROWTH LOOK LIKE?

. . . .

Question Your Thoughts and Assumptions

Stop letting yourself think, I don't do X. Instead think, Where has that thought process gotten me so far? You grow by questioning your thoughts and assumptions. If you hear yourself saying definitively, "I don't do that," take a pause and say, "Self, where has that thought process gotten you so far?"

When it comes to adopting a healthier lifestyle, too many of us get in our own way. We sabotage our own success by being married to unhelpful habits and beliefs.

Often when I suggest to someone that they modify a behaviour, like substituting eggs for their morning muffin or meeting friends for a walk instead of for a meal, their answer is an immediate and staunch "I don't do X" (eat breakfast, get enough sleep, try a particular type of fitness class, and so on). My slightly cheeky (but said with absolute love) response is this: "And where has that habit gotten you so far?"

Another way to frame the same question is to ask yourself, What story have I submerged myself in? We are all the heroes and heroines of our own narratives; we create unproductive brain propaganda–based stories to justify our unhealthy behaviour. What story have you created?

Have you created an "it's not fair" story to justify eating cake? As in, "I am saddled with terrible genetics. It is not fair. My sister can maintain her weight and eat cake." Too much cake is bad for you no matter what your weight. Life is not fair. You are an adult. Own your genetics. Stop using them to justify bad behaviour. Are you submerged in the "life is short so I deserve X" narrative? Life is short, so love yourself enough to eat nutritious food and exercise so you can make the most of your time. Question your stories, your assumptions, and your brain propaganda.

 Try my Flip It challenge. The goal is to divorce yourself from your current rules — flip what you do and don't do. If you are unhappy with your health, what you are doing is obviously not helpful or useful. Choose a time frame — maybe a week, a month — and whenever you think or say, "I don't do X," stop and ask yourself if it would be helpful to your health to flip the sentence to "I *do* X." Change "I don't eat vegetables at breakfast" to "I am going to try vegetables in my omelette." Or "I don't eat breakfast" to "I am going to make overnight oats and have them for breakfast for a week." Or "I don't do that type of workout" to "I am going to try a new workout every Wednesday for a month. If I like any of them maybe I will continue going. If not, I will go back to my old workout." Your old habits will always be there. You can revert back to steadfast habits if needed, but you have to try new things to know what will stick; how can you expect to become a healthier version of yourself if you're not willing to question your habits or beliefs and do things differently?

Actively create the healthier version of you that you want to be. The key word is actively. Adopting a healthier lifestyle isn't a passive process; you have to actively create the healthier version of yourself that you envision.

TIPS FOR ACTIVELY CREATING YOUR FUTURE YOU

- **ASK YOURSELF, WHERE HAS THAT BELIEF OR HABIT GOTTEN ME?** Stop sabotaging your own success by being married to how you always do things. Ask yourself, Where has that belief or habit gotten me? Don't eat vegetables? Become someone who does. Don't strength train? Try it. You know where your edges are — of course you shouldn't eat things you are allergic to or do something that will cause injury — but don't let yourself off the hook just because you don't love a particular food or because you don't think you are someone who goes to the gym.

- **CHALLENGE YOUR HABITS.** You can grow to love, or at least tolerate, movement, but not if you don't try. Your taste buds can adapt over time — you are probably currently at least mildly addicted to sugar and salt — but they will only adapt if you break the addiction. Eat some kale. Even seemingly healthy habits should sometimes be challenged. I find it hard to skip a run, even when I know my body needs a break from the impact. I need to learn to prioritize cross-training, because over-training leads to injury.

- **ASK YOURSELF, WHAT TYPE OF PERSON DO I WANT TO BE?** If the person you want to be has different values than your current self, decide if you can legitimately shift your value system. If yes, look around and find someone who holds those beliefs and values. Talk to them. Learn from them.

Learn to Lean In to the Fall

When you fall off of your health horse, don't just get back up; get back up with purpose, gusto, and pride that you were willing to fall in the first place. Take the opportunity to learn from the fall so that you get back on as a more informed rider. Every fall is an opportunity for growth and learning.

Traditionally, one of my most used Kathleenisms has been "When you fall off of the fitness horse, get back on as a more informed rider." Recently, I decided that the original Kathleenism — although useful — required some tweaking. The original is premised on the assumption that an occasional fall is normal — which is true; we are all human — but it doesn't express that falling is not only inevitable but can be positive.

Don't misunderstand me. I am not suggesting that you fall on purpose. But when you do fall, be proud that you are even aware of the fall, and take the opportunity for growth.

Being aware that you fell — that you deviated from your plan — demonstrates that you are mindful of your behaviour and that you have at least a semblance of a plan; noting a health choice proves that you are in the game.

To paraphrase Brené Brown — a woman I respect immensely — from her book *Daring Greatly*, the only people who don't fall are the ones not stepping into the arena of life.

Let me reiterate: I am not suggesting that you fall on purpose. Don't say,

"Kathleen says we all slip, so it is healthy for me to get drunk and then have four pieces of chocolate cake." Rather, when you make a choice that your future self will not be proud of, lean in to the fall and learn from every choice, both positive and negative. Work to understand your personal triggers and coping mechanisms so that you evolve into the healthier and fitter future self you want to be.

TIPS FOR LEANING IN TO THE FALL

- **WE EITHER GROW AND ADAPT, OR WE STAGNATE.** Ask yourself, Am I content with my health? Am I happy with how I navigate life's ups and downs? If your answer is no, then your only productive option is to grow.

- **EMBRACE THAT GROWTH TAKES WORK**; choose a goal that equates to the amount of struggle and work you are willing to put in. You can't just be okay with the result (for example, weight loss); you have to be okay with the process (for example, the work needed to lose the weight). Who your future self will be is connected to what you are willing to struggle for.

- **AS A START, CONSIDER IMITATING THE BEHAVIOUR** of a healthy and happy person who has traits and habits you would like to adopt.

All experiences are opportunities for growth and learning.

- ***ACT* TO SOLVE**. Take small steps if needed, but take steps. Don't just wish for better health. Make a plan and follow it. Health is an active process.
- **LIVE LIFE AS IF YOU LOVE YOURSELF**; work out and eat well because you love your body not because you hate it.
- **EMBODY THE KNOWLEDGE THAT YOU ARE HUMAN**. You have emotions — you are not a robot — and thus will fall off the horse from time to time. Instead of letting this reality frustrate you, frame your fall as feedback. Use the feedback to propel you forward; get up stronger and wiser. Negative emotions are not bad; they are a call to action — a way for you to understand your limitations and thus to grow.
- **FLIP YOUR MINDSET**. Buy in to the fact that health is made, not found. To be successful in your health process you need to revel in perseverance. Stop aiming to eliminate all problems and instead aim to learn to manage problems and figure out situations.

Learn — through falling — how to make choices that your future self will be proud of. Love yourself enough to demand more of yourself. Don't let yourself off the hook; when you fall get up, learn, and grow. Work to find solutions, not excuses. Or as Brené Brown would say, make your goal to "show up and be seen."

Aim to Grow but in a Way That Respects Your You-Ness

Trying to adopt a method of change that doesn't fit your personality is futile. Yes, your fittest future self can be a reality, but for the changes to stick, they have to be made on your terms.

Sure, you can twist yourself into knots and adapt to someone else's program for a few weeks, but chances are you won't be able to maintain the program over the long haul. Adopt a method of change and a lifestyle regimen realistic for you.

STRATEGIES FOR GROWING

A crucial part of adopting a healthier lifestyle is respecting your you-ness while navigating the formulation of your individual WORKOUTmix, NUTRITIONmix, and MINDSETmix. Don't worry; I will teach you how to formulate those mixes in chapters 3 through 9, but first let's answer the question, What does respecting your you-ness even mean?

Respecting your you-ness means that, as you put together your WORKOUTmix, NUTRITIONmix, and MINDSETmix, remember that success is not driven by simply finding information that fits you but also by matching the implementation strategy to who you are and how you are motivated — your you-ness.

Motivated by large, grand changes? Maybe you need to cut out sweets entirely for a month or try something more prescriptive like the Whole30 program for thirty days. Motivated by small manageable goals? Perhaps a gradual increase in your step count and being moderate with desserts might suit your you-ness. Do you

Don't try to fit a square peg into a round hole. Other people's health and diet regimens are exactly that — theirs.

work best if you combine your efforts with others? Maybe you need to join a sports team. Or are you a solo achiever? Sign up for a running race.

For example, if you know you are most successful when you implement changes gradually, try my weekly add-on method. If you like radical change, try my 180 daily pyramid method for change.

Fifteen years ago I regretted almost every health choice I made. The regret was exhausting, demoralizing, and demotivating. Now, I still occasionally regret a choice, but the older I get — and the more I become aware of what actually makes me happy rather than what I think will make me happy — the better I am at making choices that my future self will be proud of. My regrets have become fewer and further apart. I envision my health process like the stock market — as long as I am trending positive, I am happy. I don't aim for health perfection or a linear improvement. Instead my goals are three-fold: to have fewer unhealthy habits this year than last, to stay the course, and to learn from every choice I make.

WEEKLY ADD-ON. First, make a list of health habits you would like to adopt. For example, eat five or more servings of vegetables daily, drink more water, eat fewer fried foods, or cook more food at home. Next, decide which changes will make the most impact on your overall health. For example, you might hear that everyone will lose weight if they cut out alcohol. But if you hardly ever drink, that suggestion is unhelpful to your quest. You might find it more worthwhile to eliminate your three o'clock sugar binge. Last, pick one to two changes and commit to doing those for a week. After you successfully complete them for a week, maintain them and add on another change the following week. Continue to add on positive changes until you have implemented all your new healthy habits.

180 DAILY PYRAMID. As with the weekly add-on method, start by making a list of the changes you would like to make. Next, ask yourself how long you could realistically maintain all the changes. Be honest.

Let's pretend you said two days. Commit to being 100 percent disciplined for those two days, knowing that once you finish your two days you can eat normally for a day. Once you complete your two days, take your normal day, and then stick to your goals for three days. Once you can do three days, aim for four, then five, and so on. Decide realistically how often you should schedule a normal day. Once per week? Once per month?

The main point is that you need to develop an individualized MINDSETmix, your targeted motivational recipe for success. This MINDSETmix should be realistic, sustainable, and built around your unique reality, rhythms, lifestyle, and personal goals. Details on how to create this MINDSETmix can be found in chapters 8 and 9.

LET YOUR FITTER FUTURE SELF STEP FORWARD

Stop getting in your own way. The slightly ironic nature of changing your health is that you have to step out of your own way to make room for your future self. You have to create two versions of yourself: one actor and one objective observer who can step back and say, "That action or thought is not helpful — let's figure out what would be better." If you learn anything from this chapter, remember that thoughts are not facts, and acts don't have to be repeated. Just because you have always thought something does not make it right; just because you have always done something does not make it the be all and end all; and just because you have always believed something does not mean you always have to. If your old habits and beliefs weren't helpful, create new ones.

Embracing curiosity and being okay with living in an atmosphere of growth and uncertainty is crucial to the mix-making process. Becoming aware of the relevant health information to parse out the recommendations that are appropriate for your individualized WORKOUTmix and NUTRITIONmix is only one part of the change puzzle. Knowledge has to become action; you can't just *know* alternative ways to be, you actually have to be different. Turning knowledge into action requires

> Question your current values, assumptions, and habits — figure out the story you are entrenched within. Then, try new ways of being.

both a MINDSETmix — you will learn how to create this in chapters 8 and 9 — and a willingness to challenge yourself.

Step aside. Stop getting in your own way. Let your new fitter future self step forward. Health is a process, and for long-term changes to occur, you have to embrace that to get different results — a fitter future self — you can't continue to repeat the same thoughts and actions. When you feel yourself resisting a healthy change, take a moment to ask, Where has my current habit gotten me? Then figure out what new habit would be more useful. Ask yourself, What type of person do I want to be? Then be that type of person. When you want that second helping or cookies after dinner hit the pause button — make yourself pause and walk away from the situation for even five minutes so you can decide how to respond rather than react to your desire. (Pausing is a huge part of creating the future self you want. We'll come back to the pause in chapter 5.) When you want to make an unhealthy choice — like skip your workout — tell yourself, "I am not the type of person who skips my workout. I am active!"

We all — to differing degrees — make health choices we are not proud of. Don't aim to make all healthy choices all the time — that is not realistic. Instead, envision a future self that respects your genetic window and current life realities. Structure your life so that you become the person you want to be. Schedule workouts into your calendar. Prepare healthy food in advance. Know you will have moments of low motivation, so don't keep unhealthy food in the house if that will help you. Plan active outings so your social time doesn't always revolve around food.

Take charge of your own health! If you become overwhelmed, don't use fear as a reason to do nothing. Make one healthy choice. Do something — anything. Eat a vegetable; drink a glass of water; go for a walk.

Act like the future self you want to be.

Decide every day to wake up and be curious; lean in to an attitude of growth, flexibility, healthy striving, and compassion.

CHAPTER 3

Your **NUTRITION**mix: Foundations

Instead of trying to find a diet to follow, create a
NUTRITIONmix — a lifestyle — you can LIVE.

What is your ideal diet?

Well, I can tell you what it is *not*.

➡ Your ideal diet is not my eating plan ... or your best friend's or your brother's.

➡ Your ideal diet is not whatever your favourite celebrity is doing at this moment.

➡ Your ideal diet is not the current fad miracle diet.

➡ Your ideal diet is probably not even the diet that worked for you ten years ago.

Now I am going to blow your mind — even your ideal diet is not the perfect diet.

I am not saying your ideal eating mix doesn't exist but rather that you have to actively create a mix that works for you. Your NUTRITIONmix!

The perfect diet is an unproductive mirage. It just sets us up to be disheartened and discouraged. Your ideal diet mix is mutable and unique to *your* needs; it is composed of the nutritional pillars and strategies that work for you based on your genetics, lifestyle, life circumstances, and goals.

Don't Aim for Perfection

· · · · · · · · · · ·

As you may be aware by now, I have a bugaboo with the concept of "perfect" — especially when it comes to nutrition. Perfectionism, to quote Brené Brown, is the "great oppressor"; there is no such thing as the perfect anything, and the act of searching for perfection is the enemy of just getting things done! There is no one diet that will make you miraculously, instantaneously happy and thin. Every person is unique; therefore everyone's ideal NUTRITIONmix will be unique.

Instead of finding a diet to follow, create a lifestyle to live.

The key words are *finding* and *creating*. Finding is relatively passive. Creating is active. Health is an active process. A large component of motivation is a feeling of control: the more you believe that your actions have an impact, the more motivated you will be to act. You won't stick with a nutrition plan long term if it is not realistic and tailored to fit your individual needs. You have to be the author of your own life — or in this case, the author of your own diet mix.

Now, I am sure you are thinking, *Kathleen, that sounds easier said than done. The mix is a nice sentiment, but how do I actually create it?* Chapters 3 and 4 are dedicated to helping you do just that. I will give you the tools to create your unique NUTRITIONmix.

The key to creating a mix is leaning in to the concept that there are pros and cons

About 80 to 90 percent of people who lose weight on fad diets regain that weight or more. To be successful long term, you have to individualize your strategy — you have to create *your* NUTRITIONmix.

to every nutrition regimen. You have to be an educated mix maker — your health is important after all. Learn about the various nutrition options available so you can parse out the nutritional guidelines that will work for you; pick and choose the elements of different plans to create a plan that works for you, one that is individualized to your genetics, age, gender, health history, goals, and life realities. Chapter 4 outlines various nutritional regimens, including pros and cons, and who might benefit from each. I conclude that chapter with my own current NUTRITIONmix, not so you will mimic me but so you can witness my nutrition thought process — how I have created a unique nutritional tapestry woven from threads from various nutritional plans and philosophies.

This chapter sets you up for success in chapter 4. Here I offer ten concepts to consider as you read through the nutritional plans in chapter 4, as well as a breakdown of six nutrition personalities. Consider which personality — or what mix of personalities — you are. Read chapter 4 with your personality in mind so you can understand how you might interact, positively or negatively, with different nutritional programs.

 If you spend considerable time reading Wikipedia or researching your next technological purchase, consider a one-week redirect challenge. For one week consciously redirect some of your research resources to understanding your body. Make the parameters of the challenge fit you. (Are you noticing a theme?) Rules for the challenge might include allowing yourself only one fun article for every health article you read, or only after a minimum of fifteen minutes of learning about health. Time is a valuable currency — you can't ever get those research minutes back — and you only have one body. Stop spending more of your valuable energy learning about movies or researching your new car than you do on your own health. Make your body a priority!

Remember the Kathleen Cycle:

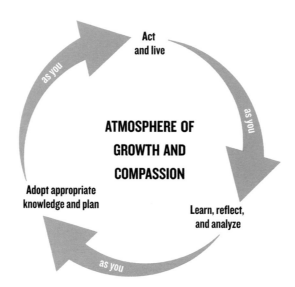

Act and live as you within an atmosphere of self-growth, awareness, and compassion; analyze and implement what you learn; and act and live as yourself with the new-found knowledge. All experiences are learning opportunities; live in such a way that you can learn and then live again (but as a more mature version of yourself).

In nutrition terms, this translates into eat, live, and act in a way that honours your genetics, life realities, and goals; learn and analyze (with compassion) information from trusted science and your own nutritional experiences; adopt appropriate knowledge and plan new strategies and goals; and act and live as you with your new-found nutritional knowledge.

Stop searching for a perfect diet and instead create the NUTRITIONmix that works for *you*! Understand your NUTRITIONmix as one component of your overall unique YOUmix.

WHY IS CREATING YOUR
UNIQUE PLAN IMPORTANT?

First, all regimens have pros and cons. The trick is to understand the pros and cons of each approach so you can parse out the elements that work for you and then create an individual recipe for nutrition success — your mix. No one diet works for every person; rather elements of different protocols might resonate with different people. Maybe the no snacking element of intermittent fasting or the balance approach from Weight Watchers will resonate. If so, those could be the first two guiding principles of your new nutrition program.

Second, not only will the nutritional fit be different from person to person, it will vary and evolve throughout each individual's life. Your fit will not look like your mom's, your favourite celebrity's, or mine. It will also not look like your nutritional fit in the past or the future.

Third — and this is a *big* one — adopting a healthier lifestyle is not as simple as finding the perfect diet and being disciplined enough to follow it. Anyone who tells you that probably wants to sell you something. Our eating habits are tied to our emotions, established habits, lifestyle, and childhood eating habits. Maintaining a healthier lifestyle long term involves figuring out the WWHH of *your* eating habits — *why* you eat, *when* you eat, and *how much* and *how* you eat. The operative word is you. You can stress eat or binge eat out of loneliness on any diet — lots of people overeat gluten-free cake and paleo treats. If you don't become aware of your eating patterns, your personal food habits will simply follow you from nutrition program to program.

Aim to understand yourself and the different approaches available so that you can put together a personalized plan. Actively parsing out elements of different regimens that work for you is not only the realistic approach but empowering and active; you own and understand your choices so you can stick with them long term.

Your Mix Cheat Sheet

· · · · · · · · · · ·

1. **FIND YOUR LINCHPIN AND BNB (BIGGEST NEGATIVE BANG) HABITS.** Pinpoint the habits that are proportionally causing you the most negative health repercussions.

2. **BE MINDFUL OF THE REPLACEMENT EFFECT.** Often, diets focus on elimination, but always ask yourself, What am I replacing eliminated foods with?

3. **ACKNOWLEDGE THAT AWARENESS BREEDS CHOICE.** Take stock of your actions, habits, and thoughts so that you can make honest choices.

4. **CLARIFY YOUR WHY.** Clarify why you are choosing a particular eating strategy. Your goals and eating strategy should mesh.

5. **LET GO OF RESENTMENT.** Tell your negative brain propaganda gremlin to take a hike.

6. **EMBRACE THAT FINDING YOUR MIX IS A PROCESS NOT AN EVENT.** Everything is feedback. You have to flail to learn.

7. **USE YOURSELF AS A RESOURCE.** Leverage what has worked and learn to abandon what has not.

8. **BE CURIOUS.** Find the balance between confidence in your self-knowledge and willingness to expand your thoughts and actions.

9. **BE OPEN TO YOUR MIX CHANGING.** Always have a plan, but be flexible. Know where you're going, but be excited to change course if needed.

10. **MAKE CONNECTIONS; BE A SYSTEMS THINKER.** Highlight the elements that cross nutritional camps.

TEN THINGS TO KEEP IN MIND
AS YOU PUT TOGETHER YOUR MIX

1. **FIND YOUR LINCHPIN AND BIGGEST NEGATIVE BANG (BNB) HABITS.**

The more an eating regimen disrupts your current linchpin and BNB habits, the more impact the change will have. Often linchpin and BNB habits are one and the same — but not always.

A linchpin habit initiates a significant spiral of either positive or negative actions and thoughts. If a nutrition regimen changes a linchpin habit, it will have dramatic effects on health. For example, let's say a diet asks you to cut out alcohol. If drinking is your linchpin habit, just the act of having one drink will set in motion other negative habits (like eating more, staying up late, and being unproductive the next day). I don't drink, so a diet that advocates cutting out alcohol would not benefit me. My mom can have one glass of wine and, while she enjoys it, the act of drinking it does not make her want more alcohol or spur other negative habits. Exercise

is one of my positive linchpin habits. If I do my workout, I am more likely to do other positive things throughout the day. As you read through the diets in chapter 4, keep your linchpin habits in mind. Use them as one lens to decide which approaches would positively or negatively affect your health.

Your BNB habits might not set other bad habits in motion, but they have a disproportionally huge negative impact on your health. For example, you might only eat after dinner once per week, but those empty calories have the potential — especially if your goal is weight loss — of negating your other positive daily choices.

If eating after dinner disrupts your sleep or makes you feel frustrated with yourself and then make additional negative choices, after-dinner snacking becomes both a BNB and a linchpin habit.

Some habits are not a BNB in their own right, but they can

become linchpin habits. For example, skipping one workout doesn't really affect my health in the long run, but I am much more likely to make negative food choices on days I don't move.

2. BE MINDFUL OF THE REPLACEMENT EFFECT.

While diets often focus on what you are eliminating — gluten, meat, carbohydrates — you must always ask yourself, Am I simply replacing the eliminated food with an alternative unhealthy habit? If one of the eliminated foods is your linchpin habit (you survive on white carbs, for example), eliminating that food group will only be positive if you don't replace it with another negative (especially if that negative becomes your new linchpin).

For example, if your goal is weight loss, you will not be successful if you simply replace baked goods containing gluten (such as cookies and cakes) with gluten-free baked goods, or alcohol (which is basically a sugar) with other products (such as candy or pop) that are also high in sugar.

If you're trying to eliminate white carbs, consider nutritionally dense complex carbohydrates, such as sweet potatoes, squash, or barley. If you're trying to eliminate alcohol, consider sparkling water, infused water, or herbal teas. If it is the carbohydrates or sugar in alcohol you care about (rather than the alcohol itself) consider replacing beer and wine with alcohol low in carbohydrates, such as vodka.

Now, if you eat a particular food to fill an emotional void — rather than the physical void of hunger — consider replacing the food with an activity. If you are eating because you are bored or sad, find alternative ways to fill that void. Go for a walk or call a friend.

Be mindful about what you are eliminating and what you are replacing the eliminated food with.

3. ACKNOWLEDGE THAT AWARENESS BREEDS CHOICE.

You can't make healthier choices if you are not aware of your actions, habits, and thoughts. Awareness facilitates choice. Why?

First, you have to be aware of

your nutrition choices to be able to make appropriate choices; if you are not, you don't have the data to choose well. I often tell my clients, "If you're not measuring, you're guessing."

Second — and this is key — when I use the word *choice* I am not simply talking about sifting through existing alternatives. Choice is about creating options and thus creating your desired future. Once you are aware of your actions, you can ask yourself, What choices can I create? Going to a dinner party? Offer to bring a salad. Always eat multiple pieces of bread at restaurants? Ask the waiter not to bring the basket or to only bring one piece. Create your options.

Third, think of awareness, choice, and the ability to say no as muscles. Your resilience — your "say no" muscle — needs to get stronger. Every time you use your resolve muscle, imagine it akin to a biceps increasing in tone and strength. Every day is a new day to flex those muscles. If you were a professional football player, you would not wait for the Super Bowl to practise a skill. Think of yourself as a nutritional athlete; practise saying no before the big event, because when stressed, you will go back to your default pattern or habit. The more you practise, the more saying no becomes your default.

Fourth, connect your choices to something meaningful — part of a larger project. Connect small choices like skipping the bread basket at dinner to the bigger picture of your health. Small choices often seem inconsequential, but they are not — they are part of reaching your overall end goal.

After reading chapter 4, regardless of what nutritional camp you decide to live in, embrace awareness. Awareness is a skill that crosses all nutritional camps. Stop guesstimating. Consider journaling your food for a few weeks. We typically underestimate unhealthy choices and overestimate healthy choices. Adopt the pause: before eating, reflect on what, why (anger, sadness, and so on), and how (standing, watching TV) you are eating. Detailed information on these and other mindset, motivational, and coping strategies can be found in chapters 9 and 10.

4. CLARIFY YOUR *WHY*.

Why you are choosing a particular eating strategy — whether for weight loss, blood sugar control, ethics, or another reason — your goals and eating strategy should mesh. For example, people often become vegetarian to lose weight and get discouraged when they don't. Many people, especially women, gain weight when they become vegetarian. I lost weight (unintentionally) when I stopped being vegetarian because I inadvertently consumed fewer carbs and more protein. I am not making a judgment on vegetarianism or health versus weight loss goals, but whatever your eating strategy, be informed and clear. Don't conflate weight with health. Have clear goals and know why you are changing your habits so that your choices align with the goal. Often goals like health and weight loss overlap, but not always. It depends on where you start. If you need to lose weight for health reasons, that is different from wanting to lose five pounds for aesthetic reasons. Be clear. Be informed and know why you are making your nutritional choices.

5. LET GO OF RESENTMENT.

Too often we let negative brain propaganda — in the form of a resentment gremlin — steer us off path. You know what I am talking about: It's not fair that I have to eat X. Why shouldn't I be able to eat X? He gets to eat X, so I should, too. If you experience these thoughts, give yourself a major talking-to. Tell your resentment gremlin to take a hike. We are all adults. Eating healthfully is something we are doing for ourselves, not something being done to us. Take responsibility. Your body is not a garbage can. Be proud — not resentful — that you get to put healthy food into it.

> Resentment is like ingesting poison to kill someone else. Being resentful over having to eat healthfully hurts only ourselves — and maybe our immediate family who have to put up with our ill health and snippiness.

6. EMBRACE THAT FINDING YOUR MIX IS A PROCESS NOT AN EVENT.

Everything is feedback. You will not create your mix overnight; expecting immediate success sets you up for failure. The learning process is part of the fun. Frame learning new nutritional habits as a *process* not an event. If you make a less-than-ideal choice, don't get discouraged. Instead, learn from the event. Think of the experience as feedback. Try not to be judgmental. Just note the circumstances that enabled the slip to occur (e.g., were you tired or sad?) and then figure out solutions. Think of your nutritional life like learning to swim. You splash around and look awkward at first — that is how you get better. The splashing is not a negative; the splashing is feedback. You can't learn without a little flailing.

As you attempt to find your NUTRITIONmix, allow yourself a few wobbles — or, in other words, some ungraceful falls off of your health horse. When you fall don't just say, "Oh well." Use the feedback as feed-forward information. Remember, creating your fittest future self happens in an atmosphere of self-growth. The process of navigating the creation of the mix is a learning opportunity; the process is in many ways more worthwhile than the product. Through navigating you learn about yourself; you learn what works and what doesn't, and you learn awareness, coping mechanisms, and forward thinking.

Remember, act and live as you. Learn, reflect, and analyze with compassion; plan and respond to new growth, all within an atmosphere of growth and curiosity.

7. USE YOURSELF AS A RESOURCE.

Ask yourself, What eating strategies have I used in the past and where have these strategies gotten me? So many of us develop a habit of jumping on and falling off the same health horse. We adopt a diet, lose weight, fall off the horse, and gain the weight back. Then we start the same process again. If you are always falling off this same horse, learn from it.

Also — a caveat — just because you have always done something doesn't mean it is the right thing to do.

To use Nora Ephron's line, "Be the heroine of your own life, not the victim."[*] Be the author of your own life. If you write a page you are not proud of — perhaps you eat a few cookies — take the positives from the page and write another draft.

———————————

[*] Nora Ephron, *Commencement address* (Wellesley, MA: Wellesley College, 1996).

If a strategy I outline resonates with you because it is what you have always done, it might actually be the worst strategy for you. We all have our unique flavour of self-sabotage. Ask yourself how you self-sabotage and where that has gotten you thus far. Leverage what has worked and learn from (but ultimately abandon) what has not.

8. BE CURIOUS.

Certainty is the opposite of growth. Honour your you-ness, but be curious about what regimens and strategies are available. If you have never tried a particular strategy, now might be the time. Mind the gap between who you are now (and the choices you have always made) and who you want your future self to be.

When you find yourself resistant to change, ask the question, X might be a big part of me, but is X serving me? For example, if being a vegetarian is a big part of your identity, but your iron and B12 are low, maybe ask yourself if adding fish once per week might be an option. Or if you always have a particular breakfast out of habit — like cereal — maybe consider trying a few different breakfast options and see if something sticks. Or if you always have popcorn at the movies out of habit, consider a herbal tea or bringing your own air popped popcorn from home.

9. BE OPEN TO YOUR MIX CHANGING.

Not only will everyone's NUTRITIONmix be different, but your mix will vary and evolve throughout

You are an adult.
Own your choices.

your life. What should be a constant is a general sense of awareness and deliberate choices regarding nutrition — what should be welcomed is a change in your specific mix of fats, carbs, proteins, food selection, portions, and strategies for success. For example, if you are relatively young and play sports regularly, your body will need you to consume more overall calories, probably with a focus on complex carbohydrates to fuel your activity. Your active, busy lifestyle might mean you don't have to worry about mindless eating. Your general awareness rule might simply be eat when hungry and drink enough water so you don't mistake dehydration for hunger. As you grow older, your activity level might decrease, which will diminish your overall caloric needs, but you might need to prioritize protein to maintain lean muscle. Since your caloric needs are lower, you might need a stricter awareness rule, such as no standing and eating.

Create the mix that works for you now but change it when appropriate. Always have a plan but be flexible. Know your destination — such

I aim to live by the rule that certainty is the opposite of growth — be blissfully expansive in your thoughts and actions.

as good health — but be excited to change course if needed.

10. MAKE CONNECTIONS; BE A SYSTEMS THINKER.

Find the threads that run through nutritional information; highlight the elements that cross nutritional camps. For example, very few nutrition camps say eat all the processed food you want. Why? By eating fewer processed foods and more whole foods, you get better nutrition. Nutritionally dense foods high in vitamins and minerals help you

Become aware of what motivates you — your nutritional personality — and your unique quirks. Honour your you-ness — and leverage it!

WWHH and You

• • • • • • • • • •

Learn to be mindful of *how* and *why* you eat instead of only focusing on *what* and *how much* you're eating. *What* and *how much* you should eat are clearly key — no one is going to adopt a healthier lifestyle or lose weight regularly eating large portions of junk and fast food — but *how* and *why* are also critical. Really, the key word is not what, why, or how, but *you*. Identify your personal danger zones, habits, and triggers. Late-night eating? Social nibbling? Fast food? Alcohol? The key is becoming mindful of your habits. Once you pinpoint your habits and trends, you can find appropriate solutions.

Ask yourself the following four questions.

➡ **What do I eat?** Fast food? Prepared foods? Foods high in sugar or saturated fats?

➡ **Why do I eat?** When I am tired? Sad? Angry? Am I a social eater? Do I eat when nervous or when trying to please someone? Or do I eat more when I'm alone?

➡ **How much do I eat?** Do I eat adequate portions? Always go back for seconds? Am I stuffed after a meal? Do I snack even when I am not hungry?

➡ **How do I eat?** In front of the TV? Too quickly? Standing up? Do I pick off my partner or kids' plates? Do I nibble off my co-worker's desk?

Identify the nutritional habit that is having the most negative impact on you — the habit that will give you the most bang for your habit-changing buck — and fix that first. Once you see the difference from one positive change, it becomes easier to make other positive changes. I call this the positive domino effect.

control hunger and learn methods of appetite control. Recognize the elements most camps share and figure out how you can adopt them and make them appropriate for you.

Part of being a systems thinker is knowing what motivates you. Know who you are. Then leverage strategies that fit you — with the goal that all your various systems work in unison. For example, many of my clients will deviate from their regimen if they feel trapped. They require choice — even if just an illusion of choice; their motivation personality is go with the flow. For them, a no treats in the house rule or you have to do X form of exercise backfires; they react to feeling penned in by skipping their workout or buying food and binging. They need to have something in the house, so if they want it they know they can have a bite. They need to have multiple exercise options and the ability to opt out. Usually when food is available they don't indulge and when they have an opt out option they don't skip. I am the opposite. I work best with nothing tempting in my house and when I consider exercise an absolute non-negotiable.

WHAT PERSONALITY ARE YOU?

One way to set yourself up for health success is to match your method of change — your strategies for success — to your personality. If you know from past experience that you respond well to set non-negotiables, set yourself strict parameters; don't set wishy-washy goals if you know that will not be motivating. If you know you rebel against strong rules, stop trying to set them. Know you. Do you.

➡ **Rule bound.** You thrive on strict, non-negotiable nutritional rules. You need lines to stay within. Too much choice makes you feel confused and overwhelmed. I identify with this personality most strongly.

➤ **Go with the flow.** You need balance and the flexibility to adapt what you eat depending on the day, the situation, and your mood. Too little choice makes you feel penned in — almost suffocated.

➤ **Small changes add up.** Making large nutritional shifts feels overwhelming. You prefer small changes. You are not motivated by overnight success — rather by a feeling of perseverance. You would rather decrease your number of desserts and increase your vegetable consumption so that slowly you feel healthier; you think of your health like drops in a bucket and eventually your health bucket will overflow.

I am a mix of rule bound, because it's right, and intrinsically motivated. I respond positively to non-negotiables and will act if science (or my mother) has taught me the action is right, but I will only adopt non-negotiable rules that mesh with my core values. Through years of practice I have learned that I respond best to strong guidelines — I am rule bound — but only if the guidelines are based in logic that is both scientific and something I believe in. I always filter every rule, no matter how right, through my personal internal value lens. I love exercise because it is a win-win-win. I can easily make daily motion non-negotiable because it is both right and connected to intrinsic motivators of energy, joy, fun, and self-worth. I love doing it and it makes me feel better after. My future self is only ever one workout away from a better mood. A few of my current personal guidelines include doing a minimum of one Pilates and one weight workout a week, always averaging a minimum of a nine-minute mile on my runs, and never eating past nine at night.

➥ **Big changes make you feel in control.** You need big changes — at least at first — to feel like you are doing something. A large jolt and fast initial results are motivating. Small changes feel too incremental.

➥ **Because it's right.** Extrinsic logical motivators (usually based in science) are enough to motivate you. You will make a nutritional change because a doctor suggests it or because a scientific study convinces you it is right. You make decisions based on logic, not on how an action makes you feel.

➥ **Intrinsically motivated.** You make changes because you feel happy, joyful, or a personal sense of accomplishment.

As you read through chapter 4, keep your personality in mind. Most people are a combination of multiple camps. The proportions shift depending on the situation.

Over time your personality will probably shift — and that is okay. Just make sure to stay mindful of the shift as it happens.

STOP BEING A NUTRITION FOLLOWER AND LEAD YOUR OWN NUTRITION LIFE

· ·

The key to long-term nutrition success is to stop being a follower. Learn the facts. Know yourself. Understand the basics of nutrition. Then, use those facts to be the leader of your own nutritional life. Create a lifestyle you can live!

As you move into chapter 4, remember these two things.

First, not only will everyone's "mix" be different, but it will also vary and evolve throughout each individual's life.

Second, not all of chapter 4 will work for you. In fact, probably more of the information won't than will. Different bits of the chapter will work for different people, and this is not only okay — it is the point. The process of navigating what works and what doesn't is what allows you to learn and grow. Some of the information is structured around the nutritional personalities I outlined, but that doesn't mean you will only find information for one personality useful. You might find that most of one personality resonates but that elements of others apply as well. One of my cardinal life rules is you never know what you will learn or what will work, so stay open and be curious. Read everything and see what works.

CHAPTER 4

Your NUTRITIONmix: Understanding the Basics

Don't just follow rules; most of us can twist any rule and make it either healthy or unhealthy. The why behind our choices, our attitude, and our dedication to our health — as well as how we interpret rules — are what matter.

In chapter 3 you considered the core concepts that will help you create your mix. By now you probably know which health personality or combination of personalities best describes you. You've bought into the mindset that creating a health mix is an active process, that you have to be the author of your own life. And you are imbued with the compassionate viewpoint that the process requires undulation for growth — creating your mix is going to be a process, not an event. All you need now is the knowledge to create your mix.

Luckily, that is exactly what's in this chapter! Before you start, ask yourself a few questions.

➡ On a motivation scale, where are you now and where do you want to be?

➡ What have you done well in the past? What strategies can you leverage?

➡ Where are you stuck? What is your limiting factor?

Work to mine the information that will increase your motivation, build on past lessons, and break through your stuck barrier.

Whatever you decide your NUTRITIONmix is, you should always have both a plan and an end goal. Use GPS as an analogy: if you deviate from your plan, figure out how to get back on track. Reroute instead of saying, "Screw it." You can reach your final healthy eating destination another way.

When you are doing the best you can and you have a C+ day, give yourself a pass. If you are working and learning, you are winning. Don't get overwhelmed by the process. Go as far as you can see … and then go further. Don't look at the nutritional mountain; decide on your first few steps. After you start you can always tweak and build your mix. But if you never start you have nothing to build on.

This chapter outlines various diets and nutritional philosophies. Read through — digest! — and figure out what elements will work for you. Start to make connections. Parse the programs to see what elements they share, such as mindfulness and an emphasis on food quality. Most regimens are more similar than you think. Use the information to establish the principles — what I often refer to as pillars — that underpin your philosophy of nutrition, that is, your unique NUTRITIONmix.

I have tried to point out who might gravitate toward each program. For example, the person whose linchpin habit is mindlessly snacking after dinner might benefit from elements of intermittent fasting. The person whose nutritional personality is balance and go with the flow might enjoy the openness of a Mediterranean diet. As you read, analyze. Reflect on the ten points from chapter 3 — particularly your linchpin and BNB habits, and your nutritional personality.

Use this chapter to gather knowledge about different diets and philosophies; know the rules of different eating regimens so that you can break them and make them your own. Finding your unique nutrition recipe — your NUTRITIONmix — is about filtering different approaches through multiple lenses: your genetics, goals,

As you read through the different nutritional programs and philosophies, keep in mind that our eating habits are tied to our emotions, established habits, lifestyle, and childhood patterns. Maintaining a healthier lifestyle long term involves figuring out the WWHH of your eating habits.

successes, and general pillars of healthy eating (such as awareness).

Fruits, vegetables, and limited processed foods are the cornerstones of healthy eating, but so are moderation and mindfulness. Instead of being discouraged by setbacks, take a long-term approach and use setbacks as learning experiences. Adopting a healthier lifestyle is a marathon, not a sprint. Stop searching for a perfect diet and instead create an eating plan that works for you.

If you are currently following a particular program — assuming it is not dangerous — and it's working for you, great! Keep at it. Adopting a healthier lifestyle can be overwhelming — having a program to follow, especially at first, can be helpful; rules can be a comforting, positive intermediate step. If you know your current self needs to dogmatically follow something like Weight Watchers, congratulations on knowing — and doing — what you need. As you follow the program, work on becoming mindful of not just what and how much you eat, but also how you eat your food and why. Once your current program stops working, resolve that your future self will not mindlessly fall off your health horse. Decide that your future self will work to figure out why the program is no longer working — what caused the decrease in motivation — and will learn from that information. Health is a process. All experiences are feedback to allow your future self to be stronger. As you mature along your nutritional path, question your regimen and habits and work toward a more expansive and flexible healthy lifestyle rather than diet.

DIET INGREDIENTS TO MAKE YOUR NUTRITIONMIX

• •

Remember, the intent of me listing various diets is not for you to find a diet. I am not laying out the pros and cons of each of these diets so that you can pick one. Instead I am offering an overview of all the options available so you can *create* an eating plan that works for you. Note, I will cite specific sources as I go, but be aware that my nutrition knowledge is based on the countless conferences I have attended over the years, knowledge absorbed through seventeen-plus years in the health field, the textbooks I used to get my degree as a nutritionist, including *Staying Healthy with Nutrition* and *The Complete Guide to Sports Nutrition*, and finally the text used within the Precision Nutrition certification. These references (and more) can be found in the appendix, Kathleen's Recommendations for Growth, Learning, and Joy.

High-Protein Diet

The common conception is that a high-protein diet is meat-based. Often, when people eat higher protein diets, they do consume more meat, but not always. As much as we try to categorize everything and water down eating styles and principles into camps, most ways of eating and nutritional principles exist on a continuum or across camps. What is "higher protein" is relative to what you are currently eating. Plus, many vegetarians and vegans are trying to eat more protein — just the non-meat variety, such as quinoa, soy products, or amaranth. Another great option is chia or hemp seeds — both offer a one-two punch of protein and healthy fats. Vegetarians who are pesco-lacto-ovo vegetarians can get protein from fish, dairy, and eggs. Fish high in healthy fats — such as mackerel and sardines — are particularly great options. If you choose to be vegetarian for moral or religious reasons but still want the benefits of eating more protein, go for it! Minimize your nutritionally vapid white foods and up your high-quality proteins. So many vegetarians are what I call *carbetarian* — they survive on mostly white carbs like pasta, toast, rice, and breads. Instead, prioritize protein and nutritiously dense foods, such as vegetables; work to become a protein-etarian or a low-carb-protein-etarian.

The positives of prioritizing protein are myriad. Protein helps with tissue growth and repair, helps the body stay satiated longer, helps decrease sugar cravings (often when you are craving sugar you are simply lacking protein), and helps minimize gorging on nutritionally vapid foods; when you eat nutritionally dense foods like protein, it's easier to stay away from empty calories like breads and sugars.

The main possible negative is digestion. Make sure you stay hydrated and eat enough fibre (or supplement with fibre) to ensure adequate digestion.

WHO MIGHT BENEFIT?

Individuals who consistently crave sugar. Often sugar cravings are due to a lack of protein. Individuals who typically feel hungry quickly after meals. Protein, along with healthy fat, is a great way to stay satiated. The go with the flow personality. Eating more protein is an umbrella recommendation with a huge amount of flexibility. Anyone with a physical lifestyle (athletes, highly active people, manual labourers) who feels their tissues do not repair adequately (a lack of tissue repair is also often tied to a lack of stage-four sleep).

WHO MIGHT NOT BENEFIT?

Those who already consume enough protein or who will use the "eat more protein" parameters to justify eating highly processed or trans-fat-filled food like chicken wings and cured meats. The rule bound personality who needs a stricter plan based on non-negotiables. For them, the recommendation to consume more protein is too vague.

Vegetarian and Vegan Diets

Vegetarianism exists on a continuum from those who eat no animal products or animal byproducts (vegans), to lacto-ovo vegetarians (no animal flesh, but hybrid products like dairy and eggs), to pesco-lacto-ovo vegetarians (hybrid products and fish).

Among the many positives, the most obvious is probably that a vegetarian diet prioritizes vegetables. (This is only a positive if you are a vegetarian or vegan who prioritizes vegetables; surprisingly many don't, surviving mostly on white carbs instead.) Vegetables are nutritionally dense and regular consumption is vital in the creation of healthy, functional bodies.

According to *Staying Healthy with Nutrition* — and many other resources I have read throughout my career — vegetarians on average have lower incidence of hypertension, obesity, high cholesterol, atherosclerosis, heart disease, and cancer — big positives! Vegetarians and vegans — in general — tend to consume fewer saturated fats and more fibre (lower fibre intake is a possible negative of many higher-protein diets, which can be problematic, since you need fibre to digest protein). For pesco-lacto-ovo vegetarians prioritizing eating more fish, a huge positive is the heart-healthy fats in fish.

The possible problems are reduced iron and vitamin B consumption and higher rates of anemia. Deficiencies in vitamin A and D are also common for vegans. Effort is, for me, the biggest negative. You can mitigate common nutritional deficiencies; you can prioritize orange, yellow, and green vegetables to get vitamin A, get vitamin D outside, and combine rice and beans to get the required combination of lysine and tryptophan. You can combine foods to get adequate protein, but this takes effort and mindfulness — skills most of us lack. The further along the continuum toward vegan, the fewer foods you can eat, and the more critical the issue of effort becomes. A final negative is hunger and sugar cravings. Protein helps you feel satiated. Inadequate protein increases sugar cravings. If you eliminate meat without finding protein alternatives, you could end up noshing too regularly on sugar-filled snacks.

WHO MIGHT BENEFIT?

Anyone with religious or ethical reasons. The rule bound personality — individuals who want to prioritize vegetables and feel they will only do so on a strict program highlighting the importance of vegetables. When adopting new habits, many people thrive on non-negotiables. Individuals who are motivated when choices and identity align. Many are more likely to consistently choose vegetables if that choice is connected to the identity shift of being vegetarian. Individuals whose linchpin habit is unhealthy meats. If you've survived on large amounts of meat in the past, your body might need a break. Often a shift from being a heavy meat eater to a pesco-lacto-ovo vegetarian is a nice balance. It allows individuals to

> There is no magic diet or food. Align your goals and choices. Prioritize knowledge and awareness. Without awareness you don't have a fighting chance.

limit fatty and fried meats (chicken wings, hamburgers, lunch meat, et cetera) and instead prioritize fish and vegetables. The big changes personality. For many, becoming vegetarian is a massive lifestyle change that has a ripple effect into all parts of life. This large change confers a sense of control and self-efficacy and can be the motivator they need.

WHO MIGHT NOT BENEFIT?

The less organized among us. Meat lovers. No one will stick to a plan they hate. You have to — in moderation — include foods you love. You can manage a plan you hate for a few weeks, but in the long term you will simply fall off the horse and end up back where you started health-wise — or further behind. As with all health choices, the individuals whose genetics do not support this particular choice will not benefit. Genetics play a huge role in how your body processes carbs, fats, and proteins.

I am constantly asked, "You eat meat?" As in, "but you're so healthy I would assume you were a vegetarian." If my journey has taught me anything it's that the presence (or lack) of meat in your diet is not the singular variable that determines whether your diet is healthy or unhealthy.

I was a vegetarian for eighteen years. At the time, it was an excellent decision — having the power to choose what I would eat at a young age was formative. Becoming vegetarian allowed me to assert independence and feel in control; feelings of control, hope, and self-efficacy are key elements of motivation and maintaining any eating style. That said, I feel stronger, leaner, and more energetic as a meat eater. But I am a way healthier meat eater than I was a vegetarian, for a few reasons: I eat copious amounts of vegetables and moderate amounts of healthy, well-sourced meats; I find eating meat protein so much easier to fit in to my diet; and I am older and can make more informed health choices. I ate lots of vegetables with both approaches.

Just to be clear (and so I don't get too much hate mail!), I am not arguing that the moral and ethical reasons for becoming vegetarian are not valid. What I am saying is, the act of eliminating any one particular food does not automatically make you healthy. For example, if you cut out sweets but replace that sugar with other forms of sugar like alcohol, granola bars, white foods, and packaged meals, the simple act of eliminating sweets will not make you healthy. I don't suggest you become a meat eater who eats bacon and chicken wings or a vegetarian who eats pasta and cheese. The meat (or lack thereof) in those meals is not what makes them healthy or unhealthy. You can be a healthy or an unhealthy vegetarian. You can be a healthy or an unhealthy meat eater. It is the big picture that matters — how everything in your day combines is key. What matters is the sum total of your decisions, not one individual rule.

Low-Fat Diet

The *low-fat diet* is an umbrella term to explain a diet that indiscriminately emphasizes reducing the consumption of fat — all types of fats including the heart-healthy omega fats. The extreme — and prevalent — interpretation is that if lower overall fat consumption is healthier, then everything labelled *low fat* is automatically healthy. Thanks to marketers and manufacturers, many people have the impression that low fat is the only thing that matters, so if something is low fat, they equate that with healthy. But for low-fat foods to taste good, they often include lots of sugar, salt, and other empty or unhealthy ingredients. Many low-fat foods are extremely unhealthy — think low fat yogurts and muffins that are high in sugar or low-fat desserts that are filled with preservatives and artificial colours.

Good Fats and Bad Fats

• • • • • • • • • • •

Good healthy fats are monounsaturated fats and polyunsaturated fats. Foods rich in monounsaturated fats include olive, rapeseed, and almond oil; avocados; olives; nuts; and seeds. An important subcategory of polyunsaturated fats is essential fatty acids, which cannot be made in your body.

That means you need to eat them. They are grouped into two series: the omega-3 and the omega-6 series. Omega-3s are especially important; they minimize post-exercise muscle soreness, improve delivery of oxygen and nutrients to your cells, enhance aerobic metabolism, and increase energy levels and stamina. Further, omega-3s are anti-inflammatory, which means they reduce inflammation caused by over-training and prevent joint, tendon, and ligament strains. Sources of omega-3 include salmon, mackerel, trout, cod liver oil, flaxseed oil, walnuts, and pumpkin seeds. Fun fact, according to *The Complete Guide to Sports Nutrition* by Anita Bean, broccoli has 0.1 grams of omega-3 per 100 grams, which is the same as one non-fortified egg.

The main positive, other than general awareness of food choices, is that if your current fat consumption is high, decreasing overall fat consumption could have positive effects on overall health. The problem is, the concept of low fat does not distinguish between good and bad fats. Healthy fats should make up between 20 and 35 percent of your total calorie intake. Most of us could use a decrease in unhealthy fats found in baked goods and fried foods but an increase in healthy fats found in olive oil and fish. Too often the label *low fat* is used to justify unhealthy choices. Most of the time when people tell me they are following a low-fat diet, it means they are eating tons of high-sugar, nutritionally vapid and processed foods such as muffins, puddings, cereals, and yogurts. In addition, chronically low-fat diets can leave you deficient in various nutrients, making you susceptible to, among other things, dull flaky skin, cold extremities, hormone imbalances, and poor control of inflammation.

WHO MIGHT BENEFIT?

There are those who might benefit from a lower-fat diet, particularly individuals whose BNB habit is unhealthy fats. If your current diet is predominately trans and saturated fats (think French fries and chicken wings), limiting fat would be a simple way to improve your overall health. Simple is good. In my experience, people often fall off the horse when a regimen feels too complicated. Individuals whose linchpin habit is unhealthy foods or who justify other negative health choices after they give into one fat-filled fast food meal might also benefit from adopting a lower-fat approach. You know the negative brain propaganda I am talking about — the "I had that burger so I might as well have wings and a few sauces as well" thought spiral. One final group who might benefit from the low-fat approach is informed consumers who are motivated by the low-fat umbrella to shop the outside of the grocery store — which for the most part will mean buying unlabelled, low-fat, fresh produce and lean proteins. These informed consumers understand

> Avoid processed foods. They are almost never healthy — no matter the label. Prioritize high-fibre, nutritionally dense foods, such as vegetables, lean proteins, nuts, and seeds.

the difference between good and bad fats, and that a lower-fat diet does not mean a no-fat diet. It means decreasing overall fat intake to within a healthy range, prioritizing healthier fats, and working to eliminate trans and saturated fats while still consuming lots of fruits and vegetables (which are inherently low fat). These informed consumers might also just say they are following a Mediterranean diet or a balanced approach.

WHO MIGHT NOT BENEFIT?

Anyone with a tendency to use dogmatic diet rules to justify choices they wanted to make anyway. At a wedding recently the person sitting beside me was eating a very large piece of cake and telling me it was healthy because it was low fat. Low fat does not mean healthy. Low-fat diets are an outmoded approach, and they were largely misconstrued anyway.

The GI Diet and Glycemic Index

The glycemic index is a ranking of foods based on their effect on blood sugar levels. The higher the number — on a scale between 0 and 100 — the faster the rise in blood glucose. A value of 100 is equivalent to consuming pure glucose.

The glycemic index needs to be differentiated from diet books that use the index, such as *The GI Diet* by Rick Gallop.* The GI diet is a method of choosing foods based on their ranking on the glycemic index, as well as their fibre and protein combination. The glycemic index is not a diet; rather, it is an informational tool (e.g., glycemicindex.com).

The index can be used as one factor when considering food choices. For example, I prioritize berries over a higher-GI fruit such as mango or pineapple; berries are relatively low on the glycemic index and are nutritionally dense (i.e., highly nutritious relative to their calorie count). That doesn't mean you should never eat mango. It means when you do eat higher-GI fruits, you should consider pairing them with a food high in fibre or protein, watch your portion, and consider them a dessert-like food (i.e., a treat).

The main positive of the index is that it is a concrete demonstration that all carbohydrates are not created equal — an important lesson for most of us. When used productively, the index fosters mindfulness, and allows for intelligent food choices and

---

* Rick Gallop, *The GI Diet*, 10th Anniversary Edition (Toronto: Random House Canada, 2011).

pairings. Plus, the index has scientific validity, and all of the books I am aware of that use the principles of the index are not based in unrealistic, fad philosophies.

The biggest potential problem is one inherent to any table, graph, or list of data; misinterpretations occur when the information is taken out of its wider context. The implication of an individual food choice needs to be understood in relation to the person's total diet, goals, and activity level. For example, it is easy to over-consume lower- and medium-GI foods when a person doesn't understand glycemic load: the amount of carbohydrate per portion times the glycemic level of the individual food — or, simply put, the quantity of carbohydrate consumed. For example, white potatoes are higher on the GI scale relative to sweet potatoes, but if you eat multiple servings of sweet potato versus half a portion of a white potato, your overall load will be higher. If you are curious about the glycemic index, don't bookmark the graph online for reference; read Rick Gallop's book (or an equivalent) to understand the larger context.

WHO MIGHT BENEFIT?

Anyone whose BNB habit is high-GI foods such as fruit juices, high-GI fruit, or white breads and pastas. Plus, anyone who enjoys research — who wants to get the big picture — or who wants a realistic, moderate, scientifically backed approach. The because it's right, small changes add up, and rule bound camps might gravitate toward utilizing the data.

WHO MIGHT NOT BENEFIT?

If you're not great at controlling your consumption of healthy foods (e.g., you easily take advantage of loopholes like the it is healthy loophole to overeat), then stay away. The big changes camp might find the changes too gradual.

Ultimately, what matters is the combined effect of everything that you eat. Thus, anyone who doesn't love having to step back and take a big picture approach will find this way of eating frustrating.

Mediterranean Diet

A Mediterranean diet consists of consuming healthy fats (in moderation), decreasing unhealthy fats, decreasing meat from land animals but prioritizing fish, and shopping regularly for fresh fruits and vegetables.

According to *Staying Healthy with Nutrition* — and the prevailing health discourse — a large positive of the Mediterranean diet is that it is associated with lower incidence of heart disease and it highlights the importance of unprocessed, whole foods. For recipes and information, consider books such as *The Mediterranean Prescription: Meal Plans and Recipes to Help You Stay Slim and Healthy for the Rest of Your Life* by Dr. Angelo Acquista.

From experience I know that the main possible problem is that for those who want to lose weight, but who already follow a fairly healthy diet or have consumed a fairly balanced diet for years, a Mediterranean diet might not be different enough. Other approaches might be required.

WHO MIGHT BENEFIT?

Anyone managing a heart condition, high blood pressure, or high cholesterol, particularly those concerned with their cardiovascular health who have intrinsic motivation — they are willing to eat better when they know it will improve their medical conditions. Anyone with the go with the flow personality — those who thrive on choice and enjoy whole, unprocessed foods, cooking daily, and prioritizing time with friends and family (the Mediterranean diet and culture centres on shared dinners). The small changes add up personality. A Mediterranean diet, for most, is not dogmatic or extreme. It obviously takes

dedication and mindfulness, but there are fewer strict rules than in programs such as the ketogenic diet or Whole30 (a strict eating regimen that includes absolutely no sugar, alcohol, or stimulants for thirty days).

WHO MIGHT NOT BENEFIT?

The rule bound personality. A Mediterranean diet can be too open-ended — many find it too directionless. The plan is not overly prescriptive, which is good if you like choice, but it can feel overwhelming if you are new to the nutrition game. People who hate fish. Those with a tendency to overeat in large groups. *Staying Healthy with Nutrition* points out that the diet emphasizes the joyous social nature of food — including savouring food while with others — which often occurs late at night. Eating late at night surrounded by the distraction of others will not be helpful for individuals who find it hard to moderate their eating within a social atmosphere.

Weight Watchers

Weight Watchers is a business. Foods are assigned points. Individuals, depending on their current weight and goals, have a set number of daily and weekly points. The goal is to stay within your point value.

A huge positive for many is the social aspect. Whether you go to meetings or join the online community, it is motivating to be accountable to someone and to know you are not alone. Members always have resources and information — either their in-person group leader or online information — to fall back on. They can ask their leader for healthy snack alternatives, family-friendly healthy meals, and new ways to stay motivated. Counting points ensures you are mindful. Mindfulness is an aspect of healthy eating that crosses all nutrition camps. Awareness brings choices, but you have to be aware of your choices to make the best choice.

A large potential problem is the tracking. For some, tracking is essential and motivating; for others tracking can seem tedious and overwhelming. Also, when allotting points, too often people choose zero- or low-point options over nutritiously dense choices, which in the end hinders weight loss. For example, someone might eat multiple pieces of fruit as snacks because they count as zero points. Fruit is highly nutritious, but if your goal is weight loss, you're better off having half the banana and two or three points of a high-quality protein. That snack might be more points, but it will keep you feeling satiated longer and has less of a negative effect on your hormones and blood sugar.

WHO MIGHT BENEFIT?

Anyone who likes community, likes tracking data, or whose linchpin habit is a lack of mindfulness around food. Anyone who likes structured balance. In Weight Watchers you can have the treats you love as long as you count the points. So, have the pizza but have one slice and have lots of vegetables throughout the day. Weight Watchers offers a unique marriage of strict rules and flexibility; this is often a good fit for rule bound and go with the flow personalities.

The small changes add up personality. Weight Watchers advocates lifestyle changes and incremental weight loss.

WHO MIGHT NOT BENEFIT?

People who find counting points frustrating. Some go with the flow people get frustrated. The big changes personality and some rule bound personalities often find Weight Watchers not enough; faster, more immediate changes are desired. People who use the rules to justify less-than-optimal nutritional choices and learn to game the system. For example, many people eat copious amounts of free fruits or eat just under a certain calorie range of a food so it counts as free, forgetting that multiple small indulgences do add up. Another way they game the system is eating because they have points left — even if they are full. If you are full, listen to your body and stop eating, even if you haven't eaten all your points. No matter what you are eating, it is crucial to learn to stop when you are full.

Macrobiotic Diet

This is a primarily vegan diet that includes occasional white fish. A main objective is improved digestion. Thus, followers consume primarily cooked foods on the premise that cooked foods are easier to digest.

Whole grains such as brown rice, rye, and buckwheat provide 50 to 60 percent of the diet. Less than 5 percent of foods consumed are raw. Few fruits and no dairy, processed foods, or animal meats are consumed. Each meal should be 20 to 25 percent vegetables, but nightshade vegetables (like tomatoes, peppers, and eggplant), avocado, spinach, and yams are not allowed. Beans, seaweeds, and pickled vegetables should be included in every meal.

A big positive is that this diet is low in sugar — always a good thing! There is no disputing the positive health implications of eliminating processed foods while prioritizing vegetables and healthy fish. Seaweeds and pickled vegetables are healthy foods often not prioritized in typical North American diets. A macrobiotic lifestyle offers individuals the chance to consume a mainly vegan diet while still eating fish — a nutritional powerhouse.

The main possible problem is a lack of variety and the dogmatic rules for rules' sake elimination of healthy foods (such as nightshade vegetables and avocado). If you have trouble digesting nightshades, eliminate them; if you don't have that problem, I see the act of cutting them from your diet akin to discipline for the sake of discipline. The same goes for the rule of eliminating raw foods. If you have problems digesting raw foods, eliminate them, but think about also addressing why this problem is occurring (the cause) versus simply eliminating the symptom (raw foods). Do you need a probiotic? Are you overly stressed? Figure out why your digestion is compromised. If you have no problems digesting raw foods I see no point eliminating them long-term. Two final possible negatives are the raw vegetables missing from this diet — veggies are yummy and nutritious — and the potential for vitamin D and B deficiency.

WHO MIGHT BENEFIT?
People with digestive distress often find the macrobiotic diet helpful, especially short term.

WHO MIGHT NOT BENEFIT?
The go with the flow personality; the lack of variety could become boring or feel stifling.

Ketogenic and Paleo Diets

The ketogenic diet advocates extremely low carbohydrate intake (ten to fifteen grams daily) and high fat consumption (75 percent of your diet). The goal is to put your body into ketosis so that it uses ketones as energy. The rationale is that the diet gives you the benefits of fasting (such as fat loss) without actually having to fast. A sample ketogenic meal might include a small portion of animal protein and butter, a small amount of green beans and butter, and a full avocado.

I know I am supposed to be neutral but — full disclosure — I would die consuming fifteen grams of carbs per day. I need more than a few handfuls of cauliflower or leafy greens.

The paleo diet — based around eating foods early humans would have consumed — also advocates fewer carbohydrates than current typical North Americans consume but allows relatively more carbohydrates than a ketogenic diet. Paleo encourages the consumption of healthy fat but relatively less than a ketogenic diet. You are not allowed carbohydrates from grains, beans, or legumes. Carbohydrates from fruits and vegetables are encouraged. A sample paleo meal might include a decent-sized portion of animal protein, green beans, half an avocado, and some sweet potato.

The main positives are that protein and fat aid satiation. Thus, lowering carbohydrate intake and increasing fat and protein intake can positively affect consumption levels. Another huge positive is that both advocate eliminating processed foods and only consuming whole, nutritionally dense foods. Typically, paleo diets are high in fibre (thanks to fruits and vegetables) and omega 3s (thanks to nuts, seeds, and high quality fish).

Possible problems include a lack of nutritional balance, especially for the ketogenic diet. The ketogenic diet is very restrictive — a bad thing if you crave freedom and balance. Most dairy (except high-fat items like butter and certain cheeses), fruit, grains, beans and legumes, starchy vegetables, and slightly sweet vegetables like winter squash, beets, corn, or carrots, and processed foods are not allowed. Carbohydrates are relatively heavy to store. You may lose weight

> If you try higher-protein or lower-carbohydrate diets, prioritize water. Your kidneys need water to support ketosis.

initially, but if you go back to your regular eating, you will gain the weight back.

WHO MIGHT BENEFIT?

Individuals who genetically can metabolize fats and proteins or, relatively speaking, have trouble metabolizing carbohydrates, and those whose linchpin habit is excess carbohydrates. Limiting carbs, especially short term, can be a positive mental reset to teach the brain it can survive without those three pieces of bread. That said, for most, the ketogenic ask of ten to fifteen grams is not sustainable. Others who might benefit include those with rule bound and big changes personalities.

WHO MIGHT NOT BENEFIT?

Anyone whose body can't metabolize fats, which is most people, or anyone who craves freedom, variety, or balance, the go with the flow personality, or those who believe small changes are the sustainable long-term approach.

Intermittent Fasting

Intermittent fasting also has the goal, in part, of bringing the body into a ketogenic state. It advocates pushing time between meals up to sixteen hours. Like most eating plans, intermittent fasting exists on a continuum; some advocates suggest eating only one meal a day; others, two meals. Some advocate a day a week where you abstain from eating. Others suggest simply elongating the time between dinner and breakfast.

WHO MIGHT BENEFIT?

Anyone whose BNB habit is mindless eating. If you mindlessly graze, spacing out meals — and thus not snacking — makes abstaining from food between meals a helpful non-negotiable.

Anyone whose linchpin habit is late-night snacking. If you commit to ten or more hours between dinner and breakfast, you can't snack while watching TV — which for many is a huge health problem. The rule bound personality and those who are motivated by large changes.

WHO MIGHT NOT BENEFIT?

The go with the flow personality or those motivated by small changes that add up. Anyone who overeats after long stretches of not eating (me after more than six hours) or those with blood sugar irregularities (like diabetes) who have been instructed to eat at regular intervals.

Own Your Choices

• • • • • • • • • • •

Be honest with yourself. Too many of us underestimate our unhealthy choices and overestimate our healthy choices or let our negative brain propaganda convince us choices are justified. Don't misrepresent reality; don't tell yourself you were hungry when really you were depressed. Figure out if you eat more when angry, sad, tired, or hurt. Don't tell yourself you only had two glasses of wine if you actually had four servings in two big glasses. The size of the glass counts! Don't tell yourself you only had one serving of dinner when you ate while cooking (this is classic Kathleen). Food counts even when it's not on your plate. If you decide you want wine, enjoy it. Own and enjoy the choice you made. Then, learn from the choice so that you can make a better choice next time. Or if you decide to make the same unhealthy choice again, fine, you only live once. But own it and understand how it affects your goals.

Food Delivery Services

Food services seem to be only growing in popularity — you can get almost every diet delivered from low fat to ketogenic. Now intermediary food delivery services — ready-made kits — are even an option. If you want to have all your ingredients freshly purchased and prepped for you, but still experience the act of cooking without leftover ingredients to throw out, you can. As a busy person I get it. All versions of delivery services diminish the time and complex planning aspects of eating well, both of which can be overwhelming.

Delivery services can be a great stop-gap — a way to learn what a balanced day of eating looks like and to get the ball rolling. Starting the health train is often the hardest part. The trick is to use the little win of the service to propel you forward and to take the time to set yourself up for success; create a plan for after the service is done.

However, not all services are created equal. They range from Jenny Craig, which primarily relies on packaged, sodium-filled foods, to locally owned services with fresh food. Make sure to research the service before ordering. Services don't teach you new habits. They give you the fish rather than teaching you how to fish. This is fine as a stopgap, but you have to use the time on the service to develop a plan of action and research healthy meals.

WHO MIGHT BENEFIT?

Those with big changes and rule bound personalities. Delivery services can represent a big shift in habits, and because meals are delivered, your choices are determined in advance.

WHO MIGHT NOT BENEFIT?

The frugal among us. Services can add up. The go with the flow and small changes personalities. Such services might limit choice and be too drastic a change for some.

The Vague "Betterness" Diet

The vague betterness diet is what I call the eat less of everything and make substitutions when possible way of healthy eating. Individuals using this approach are often a combination of the go with the flow, intrinsically motivated, and small changes personalities. Simply making substitutions makes healthy eating less expensive and overwhelming.

The concept is finding ways to tweak your existing life rhythms for maximum health returns. You can still have pasta, just have bean pasta. Have cereal, just have a low-sugar variation. Enjoy your coffee, but find substitutions for the sugar.

HEALTHY SUBSTITUTIONS

1. **WHEN HANGRY,** instead of mindlessly grabbing the nearest thing, consciously choose something low in sugar and high in protein like a hard-boiled egg. Carry healthy snacks with you.

2. **INSTEAD OF NUTRITIOUSLY VAPID WHITE PASTA,** have bean pasta, quinoa pasta, or a vegetable alternative. Invest in a spiralizer and make "pasta" with zucchini. Or bake a spaghetti squash and scoop out the stringy flesh inside. Add nutritious sauce with lots of vegetables and protein.

3. **INSTEAD OF SUGAR IN YOUR COFFEE,** try cinnamon. Cinnamon is slightly sweet and works well as a sugar substitute. And according to *Staying Healthy with Nutrition*, it also helps relieve nausea, vomiting, and indigestion; is beneficial for the heart, lungs, and kidneys; and can protect against diabetes by improving insulin's ability to metabolize blood glucose.

4. **INSTEAD OF RICE,** try cauliflower rice. Chop cauliflower until it resembles rice (you can use a food processor),

steam, then load with yummy spices and toppings. (Thanks to my awesome client Trudy for this idea!)

5. **INSTEAD OF BEING HEAVY ON THE MEAT,** try chopped mushrooms. Dice mushrooms by hand or with a food processor and replace some of the meat in your recipes with them. Mushrooms have a meaty texture; your meal will feel meat-heavy, but it will be vegetable-heavy — and yummy and nutritious.

If you crave…		Try substituting…
a sugary treat	➡	a hardboiled egg
white pasta	➡	bean pasta, quinoa pasta, spiralized zucchini, or spaghetti squash
sugar in coffee	➡	cinnamon
rice	➡	cauliflower rice
meat	➡	mushrooms
cereal, granola	➡	Hi-Lo cereal
muffins	➡	egg muffins
pizza	➡	egg pizza
ice cream	➡	protein pops

6. **INSTEAD OF GRANOLA,** try Hi-Lo cereal. Cereals tend to be high in sugar and processed ingredients. I encourage clients to have hard-boiled eggs and vegetables or chia-seed pudding with berries for breakfast. But sometimes convenience is paramount and cereals are convenient. Hi-Lo has twelve grams of protein and only three grams of sugar. It is crunchy and works nicely in Greek yogurt with berries. (Thanks to

I have been working on my mix for almost twenty years — and I still tweak it daily. It changes depending on what I'm training for, the season, my current goals, current research, and mostly my experiences. If a strategy or guideline works, I keep it as one of my pillars — one of my guiding principles. If the strategy or rule stops working — or new science conflicts with old information — I adapt my mix accordingly.

My current mix is about being aware of what I put in my body — stopping eating when I am full, for example — as well as pillars from various sources. I limit snacking and aim for a substantial gap between dinner and breakfast — thanks intermittent fasting. I eat almost exclusively from the outside of the grocery store (fresh fruits and vegetables, lean proteins, and good-quality fats), thanks to paleo and habits formed while vegetarian. When possible, I choose low- to moderate-GI foods. When I do eat higher-GI foods I eat a small portion and pair it with fibre or protein — thanks, glycemic index. For example, if given a choice I pick basmati over white rice. I eat what I love in moderation — thanks, Weight Watchers, for the balanced approach.

I use what works for me and ignore what doesn't.

Your job, when you are ready, is to parse the elements that will work for you. Take an active role in your health.

my knowledgeable colleague Dr. Kendall-Reed for this tip.)

7. **INSTEAD OF MUFFINS,** have egg muffins. Muffins are convenient but often full of sugar and fat. Egg muffins are equally convenient but also nutritious. Make a batch every Sunday and eat them through the week. Sauté vegetables and place them into muffin tins. Beat eggs and pour roughly half an egg into each cup. Bake and refrigerate for a healthy breakfast you can grab as you leave.

8. **INSTEAD OF PIZZA,** have egg "pizza." I love egg pizza. Put egg whites or a few whole eggs into a pan. Bake until firm — that is your "crust." Add pizza toppings and bake. I usually add mushrooms, spinach, and salsa.

9. **INSTEAD OF ICE CREAM,** have protein pops. In summer, I sometimes replace my post-workout shake with a yummy ice cream–esque protein pop. Blend your ingredients as you would for a shake, pour into ice pop moulds, and freeze. I usually blend ice, protein powder, almond milk, and half a frozen banana, but feel free to experiment; try cocoa nibs, almond butter, flax, or frozen berries. A client swears by almond extract — she says it makes her pops taste like cookies.

KNOW THE RULES SO YOU CAN MAKE THEM YOUR OWN

What matters is the sum total of your decisions — not one individual rule. Any rule can be twisted and made healthy or unhealthy. With very few exceptions, it is our attitude and dedication to health that matters, not any one singular rule that we follow.

Know the rules of different eating regimens so that you can break them and make them your own. Filter different approaches through the lens of your genetics, your goals, your past successes, and the general pillars of healthy eating. If being vegetarian is your goal but you don't want to say no when at someone else's house, be a vegetarian except when a guest. If you want to be a vegetarian who minimizes nutritionally vapid white foods while prioritizing non–meat-based protein, go for it — be what I would call a low-carb-protein-etarian.

What it comes down to is that you are the artist of your own life, and that life includes your nutritional choices. Actively create a lifestyle and NUTRITIONmix that works for you.

As you work to create your health mix, remember four things.

First, have compassion for yourself. You are human. As humans we have the privilege of being wonderful, imperfect beings. Adopting a healthier lifestyle, like all of life, is about growth; if you were perfect, you'd have no place for growth.

Second, when it comes to your nutritional choices, it's the big picture that matters — the sum total of your decisions. With few exceptions, it is not one single rule that makes the difference; rather, it's the aggregate of all choices.

Third, your intentions matter. Let me state that again for dramatic effect: The intention behind how you use a rule matters. In Brené Brown's book *Braving the Wilderness*, she uses the image of fire to illustrate the importance of intention, stating that fire can either feed you and keep you warm, or burn your house down. The same act, depending on the intention and parameters, can have drastically different outcomes. For example, on Weight Watchers, are you using the fruit-has-no-points rule to entice you to not eat cake? (A positive intention.) Or are you using the free fruit rule to justify stuffing yourself with mango when you have already had three helpings of dinner? Most of us can twist any health rule to become healthy or unhealthy, so instead of adopting a rule, adopt the intention to be aware, productive, and healthy. Our attitude and dedication to our health — thus how we interpret rules — are what matter.

Aim for healthy striving rather than perfectionism. Instead of trying to be perfect and find the perfect diet, put together your unique NUTRITIONmix.

Fourth, creating your mix is a gradual process; your norms must change over time. I was not born craving healthy foods. While I still love chocolate, I now see it as a special treat and not something for daily consumption. Give yourself time to adapt and grow.

Think of your nutritional journey as analogous to sitting on a swivel chair. When you are making choices that you are proud of, you are sitting forward — the chair is stable. Making a less-than-ideal choice is equivalent to swivelling. Swivelling is normal; we are human and inherent to being human is some swivelling. The mission is not to stay robotically still — that is unrealistic since we are not robots. The mission is to recognize that you are swivelling as immediately as possible and then to bring yourself back to centre. If you swivel and mindlessly grab food off a co-worker's desk, don't think, *Oh well, I might as well have more* (thus swivelling further). When you swivel, bring yourself back with compassion; note the swivel, figure out what environment encouraged the swivel, and then work to implement strategies to avoid future identical swivels.

I am not saying to never have a treat. Savouring a small portion of something you love once in a while is not swivelling. Swivelling is mindless consumption your future self will not be proud of.

Throw off the shackles of perfection, and aim for healthy striving; if you're working, you are winning.

CHAPTER 5

Preparing for Your WORKOUTmix

Fill your health toolbox with fitness-related information, tools, and strategies; develop the skills to navigate the fitness landscape — and individualize all information — like a pro.

Chapters 3 and 4 were dedicated to finding your NUTRITIONmix. Now — drum roll please — we prepare to find your WORKOUTmix. As with the creation of any individualized "mix," finding your WORKOUTmix involves parsing the relevant fitness information and strategies that work for you. Yes, I know … déjà vu. Put another way, over the next three chapters your mission is to codify an individualized fitness philosophy, program, and possibly even language using a unique lens forged from your life realities, your goals, your genetics, and your value system.

METAPHORMIX

First, a quick insight into the world of Kathleen. My partner, James, often teases me (lovingly) about my over-reliance — his word not mine — on metaphors, not to mention my propensity to mix them. If you have noticed my love of a good mixed metaphor and wondered if I am aware of this idiosyncrasy, know that I am well aware. A good metaphor fills me with joy — and creatively mixing metaphors and making them my own puts a smile on my face. I am a big believer in both knowing the rules so you can break them and — possibly more important — doing you. I am the metaphor queen — and in my own book I am okay with that.

How will finding your WORKOUT-mix unfold? In this chapter I briefly outline the four fitness personalities — gym bunny, competitive athletic gym bunny, time-crushed multi-tasker, and homebody — discuss the importance of the pause, explain the three pillars that need to underpin your WORKOUTmix, and provide a fitness dictionary of sorts. The dictionary, or more aptly the 411 of fitness, is a list of basic information that all mix makers should know and it includes training guidelines and terminology. The goal of the dictionary is to allow all readers to, more or less, start their analysis on a level knowledge field.

Chapter 6 offers the pros and cons of myriad different workouts — everything from various fitness classes to pyramid sets to running or training for a road race or triathlon. Don't worry, I also offer tips on which personalities typically gravitate toward each. The goal? Leverage the information provided within this chapter to analyze which of the fitness plans in chapter 6 should — or shouldn't — be in your WORKOUTmix.

THE FOUR FITNESS PERSONALITIES

We are all a mixture of the four fitness personalities and the proportions of each are — and should be — fluid depending on our current life situation. For example, let's take a competitive athletic gym bunny forced into a transition. Traditionally, this bunny has primarily been a gym goer and extremely sedentary at work. Recently the gym bunny's doctor informed him that sitting is affecting his posture and overall health. He has had to become a gym bunny with a touch of time-crunched multi-tasker; he works out daily but also sets an alarm to remind him get up hourly to walk around, and he keeps a foam roller at work to do posture exercises. Evolution is good. Change is good. Becoming the future self you have always wanted to be requires change.

I introduced the four personalities in *Finding Your Fit* and outlined one specific program for each personality. How are the next 2 chapters different from the information provided there? Think of *Finding Your Fit* as Kathleen giving you a fitness fish. Here I am teaching you how to catch your own custom fitness fish. The next two chapters give you the tools

to be an educated mix maker so you can codify fitness information — from this book and discourse-wide — based on your personal realities.

As you read about the different workout modalities in chapter 6, attempt to have an unbiased lens; disentangle yourself from fitness PR and mythology. You might be surprised by how often people get swayed by fitness PR and urban legends; I wish I had a dime for every time someone has told me, "I have to run; it's the 'best' workout for burning mega calories." Sure, running burns calories, but those calories are moot if you'll do anything to avoid your workout, or if running leaves you injured and incapable of being active.

The fitness industry is just that — an industry. Companies will try to court you — that's their job. It is your job to be discriminating — to figure out what works for you. Yes, obvious advice; but we are often so consumed with novelty that we dismiss the wisdom in the obvious.

I think of picking a workout like dating. My mom always told me growing up, "Kathleen, just because a boy wants to date you does not mean you want to date him.

Do what is best for you — not him." It was my job to be discriminating and to pick the boy that worked for me, not say yes to a date to be nice. Same goes for picking a workout plan. It is a company's job to make their modality or product look enticing — they want you to spread positive hype and purchase their product — but you don't have to do anything to be nice or because it is the *it* workout. Not all pieces of equipment or modes of training are appropriate for all people. Not only do all workout styles and programs have pros and cons, but — as I always tell my clients — the pros of the best workout are moot if you can't actually make yourself do the workout. Your mission is to read through the pros and cons of each workout and make the analysis relative to you. Don't just consider if the workout is theoretically best but if the pros suit you. Ask yourself if you will actually do the workout.

WHAT PERSONALITY ARE YOU?

If you enjoy being with others, thrive on friendly competition, find designated workout areas — like the gym — motivating, or require different equipment and variety to stay into your workout, you are probably primarily a **GYM BUNNY**. If you identify with all of the above but particularly with being competitive or training surrounded by others, then you are probably primarily a **COMPETITIVE ATHLETIC GYM BUNNY**. You enjoy the structured nature of the gym, as well as friendly competition and athletic activities. If you consistently feel too busy to work out — pulled in a million different directions by your family, friends, and work — and can't contemplate getting yourself to the gym or a structured exercise class, you are a **TIME-CRUNCHED MULTI-TASKER**. At least for now, life has to be your gym. If you hate the vibe of most gyms, dislike working out in front of people, or hate wasting time getting to and from the gym but still want an intense workout, then you are primarily a **HOMEBODY**.

Remember, your personality is mutable — and *your* fittest future self personality might be very different from that

I am a mix of a gym bunny (lifting weights and trying new fitness classes or methods of training keeps me motivated) and a competitive athletic gym bunny (I love running and competing in triathlons). My adaptability personality is a combo of rule bound, because it's right, and intrinsically motivated. I respond positively to non-negotiables such as moving daily and having vegetables and a high-quality protein at every meal. However, the non-negotiable has to be rooted in something I know is right — science or a core value my mother instilled in me. I filter every rule through my internal value lens. Once I know, both intellectually and kinesthetically, that something has value, I am intrinsically motivated. For example, being active and prioritizing sleep makes me feel well; thus, it is easy for me to make both non-negotiable. My future self is only ever one workout and one sleep away from a better mood and rational thought.

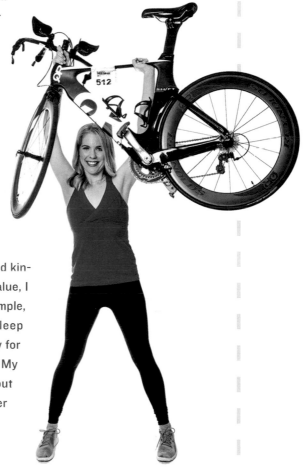

Building Your Healthy Lifestyle Muscle

· · · · · · · · · ·

Yes, staying true to your workout plan is frustrating. I get it. This health thing is not easy. If it were, the fitness field would not be a billion-dollar industry. Just remember what we discussed in chapter 3: You have to develop the muscles needed for a healthy lifestyle. Think of resilience, awareness, and the ability to say no to negative brain propaganda as muscles you are trying to strengthen. So far you have spent much of your life letting those muscles atrophy. Thus, it is unrealistic to expect them to be strong — and unrealistic expectations are the seeds of discontent and frustration. You have to work at building the muscles. Building strength takes time and dedication, but the struggle is worth it. Your health is important. Once the muscle is stronger, it will be easier to say no to unhealthy choices; healthier choices will start to feel like the norm. It is always easier to keep up than to catch up.

of your current self. That is a good thing. Change means growth. Growth is good. For example, maybe you want to work out at a gym, but you are currently too self-conscious. No problem. Your current self can work out at home knowing that taking steps to be active will allow your future self to feel strong and self-confident enough to get to the gym.

We all have to start someplace. I started doing workout DVDs at home. Give yourself permission to start at the bottom of the mountain. Take baby steps. Those steps are the only way you will eventually get to the top of the mountain. Remember, go as far as you can see … and then go further.

IN THE PAUSE

As you read through the different workouts in chapter 6, embrace the power of the pause. The pause allows for appropriate health responses. I discuss in detail the importance of appropriate responses in chapter 10. Until then, after reading each workout plan or training regimen, take a moment to reflect and ask yourself the following questions.

AM I REACTING OR RESPONDING TO THIS INFORMATION?

Reacting is emotional. Reacting is knee-jerk. Responding is allowing for that pause — creating a space between being stimulated and responding to ensure the response is positive and productive. If you realize you did react rather than respond, take a moment to reflect and dig deeper. Ask yourself, Am I reacting out of fear? Ego? Am I reacting because of a childhood memory of body shame and hate?

To create your fittest future self you have to be open to growth — and growth is made possible through a combination of curiosity and honesty to yourself.

Don't sanitize your past struggles. Let's say you have a knee-jerk "I would *never* do that" response when reading the information on how to train for a race. Ask yourself why? It is one thing to decide running is not for you based on a legitimate understanding that running is a physiological contraindication — because of past injuries or arthritis, for example. Now, on the other hand, if your reaction was fear based (you think you won't be able to finish) or you have pushed down a traumatic moment from your past when you were shamed for running, the emotional reaction might be the very reason to *try* training.

Work with that fear — rather than sanitizing it — to move forward. Use the fear as a jumping-off place for curiosity. Try running. If you hate running you can always stop. But don't let fear hold you back. Try new things. If you don't end up liking a workout — no problem. Your dislike is just feedback. No one died.

That said, don't let ego unproductively influence you in the polar opposite direction. You don't have to try everything to prove to yourself you are not afraid. Appropriate apprehension is just plain smart. Not every workout will be appropriate for everyone — and that is okay. A new workout or goal might seem novel and shiny, but if you know you *always* get injured when you run, training for a triathlon might not be for you. Embrace the pause. Use it to ask yourself, Would trying this workout make my future self happier, healthier, and more productive? How you feel by not trying something is also informative. Feedback is not good or bad; it is just feedback. Feedback is nourishment for your psychological growth.

Analyze the information in chapter 6 using both objective markers *and* your emotional reactions. Remember, mind the gap between who you are now (and thus the choices you have always made) and who you want your future self to be.

COULD EMPLOYING THIS WORKOUT, PIECE OF EQUIPMENT, OR FITNESS CONCEPT RESULT IN A LITTLE WIN?

Amass as many little wins as possible. Any little win — no matter how small — has the potential to propel you in a positive

 I challenge you for one week to note two less-than-ideal health choices per day and reframe them as growth experiences. Remember, all experiences are feedback. Finding your WORKOUTmix is a process, not an event. Your mix will not be formed overnight. The learning process is part of the fun.

How do you do this? Every night highlight two less-than-ideal choices you made during your day. Instead of judging them as bad, use the information to decide what your future self would want you to do next time. For example, if you quit halfway through a workout, figure out why. Did you go to work out hungry and thus not have the physical energy to continue? If so, pack healthy afternoon snacks. Did you overestimate your fitness and thus have to quit because the workout was inappropriate? If so, consider a more progressive build. Did you let a friend drag you to a workout you knew you would hate and thus give up halfway through? If so, resolve to find workouts you like better or learn how to say no. When you have a fitness wobble — they will happen so expect them — simply learn from the experience and then figure out solutions for future you.

direction. Is this element one key to better health? I am not saying to ignore your less-than-ideal choices. Rather, instead of berating yourself over them, note them as opportunities for growth while *also* highlighting all your daily little wins so that each little win has the potential to inspire an upward positive health spiral. A little win could be as simple as taking the stairs rather than the elevator or doing an extra workout in a week.

Let's take a sample morning. You wake up and have a glass of water before your coffee. Note that. You replace your daily muffin with a few almonds and an apple for breakfast. Note that. You prep and remember your workout bag. Note that. You take the stairs instead of the escalator at work. Note that. With those four small — and simple — changes you have noted four positive choices before nine o'clock. Use noting these choices to water a positive internal state — if you feel good about yourself, you are much more likely to then also go for a walk at lunch and complete your evening workout.

IS EMPLOYING THIS WORKOUT STYLE, CONCEPT, OR PIECE OF EQUIPMENT REALISTIC FOR ME? WILL EMPLOYING THIS WORKOUT STYLE, CONCEPT,

OR PIECE OF EQUIPMENT HELP ME TO ACHIEVE MY LONG- AND SHORT-TERM GOALS?

A workout could have countless pros, but if the program will not help you fulfill your goals, then the pros are moot. If the workout results in an injury or makes you feel shame or regret, then the pros are moot. If you hate the workout and won't do it long term, the pros are moot. Clarify your long- and short-term goals so that you know what you want your future self to be doing. Pick the strategies that will help you get there.

Clarify your *why*. As I said in chapter 3, be clear about why you are acting; your ultimate goals should underpin how you pick appropriate actions. Why are you doing what you are doing? Do you want weight loss? Muscle gain? Improved energy? Improved mental health and well-being? To fight against myriad conditions such as osteoporosis, diabetes, and cardiovascular disease?

Make sure your goals are *realistic* and *specific* — otherwise you are making wishes not goals. Have both short- and long-term milestone markers. Let's say your long-term goal is to lose twenty pounds and complete a family cycling trip. Your process might be as follows.

Read through the fitness options I outline in chapter 6, and pick strategies that will help you reach both your long- and short-term goals. Make sure to break your long-term goals into weekly or short-term goals. For weight-loss goals break your total loss down into smaller chunks — for example, say, "I want to lose twenty pounds and an average of four pounds per month." For performance goals flesh out the details. For example, don't just say "biking." Be specific — maybe your goal is bike intervals once mid-week and one longer cycle on the weekend. In terms of mindset, try to frame every daily small accomplishment as meaningful in and of itself. When you want to skip your ride say, "Self, this workout might seem like nothing, but it is significant. Biking is what will help me be strong enough to go on vacation with my family. My future self will be *so* frustrated if my entire family can go and I have to sit in the bus." Connect your choices to something meaningful — make every small choice part of a larger project.

DOES THIS PROGRAM, CONCEPT, OR PIECE OF EQUIPMENT ALIGN WITH MY VALUES?

Make sure your training plan aligns with your values. For example, if family togetherness is important to you, don't aim to go to the gym five days a week at dinner time — you will just end up ditching the gym to be with loved ones. Instead, harness and respect your value of family. Be active with them, work out at home after dinner, or do body-weight exercises as you watch your kids play sports. Or get your family involved in making dinner so you can do a shorter gym workout a few times per week and come home to a cooked meal. (You can do the dishes!)

As always, be curious and remember that failing is just feedback! If you try a workout and it doesn't align with your values, reroute and figure out another way. That said, hold yourself accountable. Don't just say "oh well" when something does not go according to plan — especially if you strayed from your value system. Yes, be prepared to fall and get up and learn, but also make sure that you are striving to be all in — to make choices you are proud of. The only time I am truly upset by an action is when I know that I let negative brain propaganda convince me of something that does not actually align with my value system.

BODY DEBT AND BODY CREDIT

There are a number of fitness goals that are fairly common: weight loss, training for a running race, and toning. If those work for you, great — but consider making one of your long-term goals getting out of body debt through amassing body credit. Body credit is each individual's level of overall health — their body's unique ability to resist physical stress. It is the body's level of energy, vitality, and physical resilience. Amassing credit and getting out of debt is one of my favourite long-term health goals because it allows for each individual to take unique, specific steps while also acknowledging the long-term and multi-layered nature of health.

Here are some activities that accumulate debt: unhealthy habits such as eating to excess, being overweight, being inactive, not sleeping enough, having poor posture, sitting too much, eating too many preservatives, and drinking too many sugary drinks instead of water.

Here are some activities that amass credit: stretching, eating well, sleeping, allowing for appropriate recovery between workouts, staying hydrated, and being appropriately active. Everyone's body credit fluctuates throughout their life — but one is either accumulating credit or accumulating debt. Age and genetics predispose people to a certain level of credit and help to determine how quickly credit replenishes itself, but everyone should always be working to accumulate credit and decrease debt.

BUILD YOUR THREE PILLARS

An appropriate WORKOUTmix includes three health pillars: strength (think push-ups, free weights, et cetera), cardiovascular (think running and biking), and stretching and mobility (think yoga and various static stretches).

As you codify your mix, make sure to include all three pillars of fitness: strength

A Rose by Any Other Name

• • • • • • • • • • •

What does Shakespeare have to do with fitness? I have decided on certain names for the three pillars, but there are multiple alternative terms floating around. For example, what I call strength someone else might label toning, conditioning, body-weight strength, or resistance training. What I call cardiovascular work could be labelled sweat session or aerobics. What I call stretching and mobility might be labelled dynamic mobility, flexibility, self-care, self-massage, foam rolling, or flow. As long as you are fitting in all three pillars, call them whatever you like!

and cardiovascular workouts, and mobility and stretching. (Don't worry. Chapter 6 outlines which workouts belong to which pillar.) The three pillars complement one another — *all three* are needed for overall health and wellness and injury prevention. For example, running will strengthen your cardiovascular system (strong heart and lungs), but the high-impact nature of the activity means that strength training and mobility work are a must. Plus, cardiovascular work, relatively speaking, doesn't build lean tissue. Strength work helps runners stay injury free, increases functional strength, and increases lean tissue (a few of lean tissue's many benefits

include increasing metabolism, helping with weight maintenance, and improving blood sugar control). Stretching and mobility work — among other things — improve functional range of motion (e.g., runners whose hip flexors have become tight post-run don't strain their backs when they're reaching for something).

Feel free to recruit multiple personalities to get the job done. For example, if you do cardio and strength at the gym, but stretching post-workout seems impossible, be a gym bunny for the first two pillars but a time-crunched multi-tasker for stretching. Piggyback your stretches onto a non-negotiable, such as watching your kid's athletic endeavours — bring a mat and stretch on the sidelines. Don't get overwhelmed; figuring out what works for you is a process. If initially you can stretch for three minutes a day and your goal is ten, appreciate what you are doing now while strategizing how to meet your goal.

PUTTING YOUR PROGRAM TOGETHER: THE 411 ON FITNESS

A *rep* (or repetition) is the act of going one time through an exercise. If your program calls for one set of fifteen reps of a squat, you need to squat fifteen times.

One *set* is the completion of all designated reps. Meaning, you have done one set of the above squats after finishing the fifteen repetitions.

Typically, we do multiple sets of every exercise. Each set is separated by a rest period. To complete three sets of fifteen reps, you would do one set, rest, complete another set, rest, then finish your final set.

I suggest using a *repetition range*, such as twelve to fifteen reps, rather than a specific rep goal (like fifteen). Start by aiming to complete the lower number. As you get stronger, aim to complete the higher number.

In time-based training, you aim to fit in as many reps as you can for a set amount of time. One example is AMRAP training, which stands for "as many rounds as possible." For more examples see chapter 6.

Don't work the same muscle group on consecutive days.

Don't do high-impact intervals like sprints two days in a row. This is especially true for beginner and intermediate exercisers.

Don't underestimate the importance of *recovery*. Exercise is only a positive stress on the body if you give it the tools it needs to recover. Stay hydrated, sleep, eat well, and do daily body self-care activities like stretching and massage.

Do complex, multi-joint exercises first. For example, do squats before bridges.

Beginners should only do two sets. As you progress, complete a minimum of three sets.

To elicit a particular training effect, the weight you use has to be appropriate for the reps completed. For example, eight to ten is considered a *hypertrophy* (or mass-building) rep range. If you could do twenty reps, but stop at ten reps, you will not build mass. Lifting a weight for eight to ten reps will only create hypertrophy if you lift a weight that you can realistically only lift for eight to ten reps.

Progression is key. I suggest beginners lift a moderate weight for twelve to fifteen reps. As you progress, use a heavier weight or manipulate reps, sets, rest periods, exercises, and even tempo. Try lowering and lifting for two counts, or lowering for four counts and powering up.

Don't forget to breathe. Don't laugh! This may sound obvious, but it is fairly common.

Don't be afraid to be aware of your body after working out — especially if the workout was new. Some positive pain or muscle soreness should be expected. However, negative pain — nerve pain, numbness, sharp stabbing, and so forth — is an indication that the workout is too aggressive or your form was incorrect. Do not push through negative pain and don't replicate a workout that causes negative pain. Seek professional guidance if you find your workouts are typically causing you negative pain.

If you have appropriate post-workout soreness, consider an *active recovery* session of dynamic stretching or light cardio such as walking or using the elliptical. Moving in a nice light way promotes blood flow.

Be mindful not to assert your *aspirational goals and habits* rather than your *lived habits,* values, and patterns. We say things like, "I go to the gym three times per week," when really that means "I *try* to go to the gym three times but usually only go twice." Become aware of what you actually do, not just want you want to do. Once aware of your choices and habits, use that knowledge to create your desired future. Choice is not merely about sifting through existing alternatives. You have to create options. If you know you always skip your workouts on Fridays because you want to do something social, plan to work out Friday morning. If you notice a pattern of Thursday night work events derailing your workout plans, make a standing Thursday walking lunch date with a colleague. That way if the workout is missed after work, at least you have moved during the day. Use awareness to create clear, realistic goals. In *Finding Your Fit* I refer to this as *making goals not wishes.*

The training variables that are most typically manipulated are referred to as the *FITT principle*: *frequency* (how often you train), *intensity* (how hard you work), *type* (what you do), and *time* (duration of the workout). A good rule of thumb to avoid injury and burnout is to manipulate only one of these variables at a time. If you increase your intensity (maybe you do intervals), don't also up the duration and frequency of your workouts at the same time.

As for frequency, remember to adopt the mindset that *something is always better*

Key Rules for Codifying Your Mix

• • • • • • • • • • •

1. **ACTIVELY FIND THE MIX** that works for you — creating a mix is *not* a passive process.

2. **BE CURIOUS AND GET INFORMED** — certainty is the opposite of growth.

3. **LEAN IN TO EVOLVING** — not only will your mix be unique to you, it should vary and evolve throughout your life. Learn about yourself so your mix can morph as needed.

4. **EMBRACE GROWTH.** Have plans and goals — but be flexible. Know your destination, such as good health, but be excited to change course if needed. When you swivel or veer off path, simply reroute; decide why you swiveled then use that information for reinvention. Think of every health choice as nourishing feedback.

5. **DO YOU.** Not every piece of information or strategy I provide will work for you. Not only is that okay, that is the point; it is the process of navigating what works and what doesn't that allows you to learn and grow.

than nothing. Start by simply embracing daily motion, no matter how small. Once you have embraced motion, then you can tweak your program.

Ideally you are aiming to complete the following:

- a strength workout (pillar 1) two to five days day per week depending on muscle group splits (for example, either do full-body workouts twice per week or legs and shoulders one day, chest and back one day, and arms and core another day)

- a cardio workout (pillar 2), such as walking, cycling, or running, that gets your heart rate between 60 and 85 percent of its max three to five days per week for twenty minutes or more
- daily stretching, massage, foam rolling, and other methods of self-care (pillar 3)
- ten thousand steps per day

Remember, these are ideals — as in eventual goals. Don't get overwhelmed; that is not productive. Work up to these weekly workout goals. Health is a process not an event.

A FINAL GALVANIZING THOUGHT: REFRAME FEAR AND ACT

Now, if you're thinking, I have always wanted to try workout X, but I have always been afraid, tell yourself to give fear the finger. Reframe fear. Instead of letting fear get in your way, say to yourself, "Fear stands for face everything and rise." If you have always wanted to try rock climbing, *do it*. If you have always wanted to take a dance class, *do it*. If "face everything and rise" doesn't resonate, try telling yourself that fear is only false evidence appearing real; fear is merely brain propaganda unless you give it the power to become real. If you tell yourself you can't do something — and then you don't do it — you have created a self-fulfilling prophecy. Try the workout. If you don't like it, or if it ends up being too challenging, then no problem. Use that as feedback. Maybe try it again in a few months.

Or don't. File the experience as a lesson learned. All experiences are just feedback.

I am not arguing you will — or should — give fear the finger every day. As a goal, that is too exhausting. But be proud of the moments when you do stand up to your negative brain propaganda. On days you give into the propaganda — you swivel — no problem. Be aware enough to note the swivel and bring yourself back to the centre with compassion. Remember, swivelling is normal. We are all human and we all swivel. What matters is that we take note, understand what happened, and implement strategies to avoid the same swivel in the future.

The most important thing to remember is that creating your fittest future self is possible — it just has to be on your terms; harness your personality and the power of the pause to curate the information with chapter 6 into a unique and realistic WORKOUTmix. Parse the fitness classes and workouts described to decide which will form each of your three pillars. Then *act*.

The only moment that you have control over is this moment. You can't control the past, and the only way to influence the future is through *this moment*.

Remember the Kathleen Cycle:

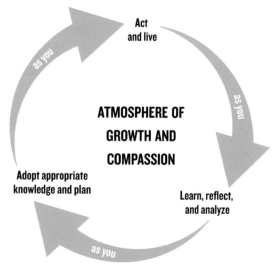

Now ... get excited! It is officially time to find your WORKOUTmix.

CHAPTER 6

Finding Your WORKOUTmix

Become a knowledgeable mix maker;
be active, curious, growth-oriented, and flexible.

Are you ready to codify your WORKOUTmix? I am hoping the answer is, hell yes!

Remember, your aim is not to pick a workout. Instead, use these chapters as a tool — a vehicle for learning how to learn about fitness. My goal is for you to be able to decide, regardless of the situation or medium, what fitness information is worth implementing and what should be filed under another life … for someone else.

You may have heard the aphorism "however beautiful the strategy, occasionally you have to look at the results."

Regardless of whether your favourite celebrity or best friend — or a scientific study, for that matter — states a particular workout plan is the "best," if the plan does not elicit the results you desire, then it is not the right plan for you.

Also, keep in mind that your WORKOUTmix needs to include all three pillars of fitness — strength, cardiovascular,

Figure out you. Do you.

Mind the gap — with non-judgmental feedback — between where you are now and where you want to be.

and stretching and mobility — but *how* you build the pillars is up to you. Maybe you do Pilates on the weekend when you can make it to a class (which falls under both the mobility and strength training pillars) and you run three times during the week out of convenience (which covers your cardio pillar). Be creative. Use multiple fitness personalities and techniques to get the job done.

Filter all information through the injury lens. If you are chronically going through the injury-recovery-injury cycle, or if a specific activity consistently causes you negative pain, use the information as feedback. Being injured is an opportunity to learn what does not work for your body. Think of an injury as your body's internal circuit breaker. Your body is telling you to stop. The activity — either in duration, intensity, frequency, or form — should not be part of your mix. You need to fix your form; decrease your frequency, duration, or intensity; increase recovery; or

eliminate the activity all together. Listen to your body.

Keep your *personalities* in mind — and I purposely use the plural. You live in a combination of camps. I feel a Harry Potter reference is appropriate here. Think of yourself as Harry. The Sorting Hat may have placed him in Gryffindor, but as readers we know he had elements of other houses within him. Your personality mix will shift depending on the situation — and over time. Personality shifting is good — evolving is good — just stay mindful as the shift happens so you can adapt your mix accordingly.

Ask yourself these questions, then choose things from each pillar that align with your answers:

- How much time can I realistically dedicate to fitness? (Remember, make goals not wishes.)
- Where and when is it realistic for me to train? (You might like going to a gym, but if being a homebody is realistic, start there.)
- Does my plan include all three pillars? If not, how can I rectify that?
- Is there anyone who might join my fitness quest as moral support,

an accountability buddy, or an exercise buddy?

- Who might derail my success? How can I mitigate that influence?
- What activities do I enjoy? How can I do what I like?
- Where do I waste time? Can I reallocate any time?
- When have I been most successful accomplishing my fitness goals? What habits did I employ? How can I leverage those habits?
- When have I been the most unhealthy? How can I avoid those situations?

Live life as a GPS — reroute as needed. Whatever your mix, always have both a plan and an end goal. When you deviate from your plan, figure out how to get back on track. Instead of saying "screw it" and letting one unhealthy choice snowball, say "reroute"; reach your final health destination another way.

Fitness on the Go

• • • • • • • • • •

When you travel, consider using the opportunity to sample different fitness classes. Trying something new is motivating. And finding the studio allows you to explore the city. Set yourself up for success; book the workouts before you go. I plan my workouts before leaving — the process keeps me accountable; I would never forfeit my money by not showing up. I especially love sampling classes in London and New York because often a few months after I try something new, the class debuts in Toronto (my home base).

THE WORKOUTS

Running or Training for a Running Race

PILLAR: CARDIOVASCULAR

Running is a fantastic full-body, do-anywhere, efficient, effective, and accessible — not to mention exhilarating and highly addictive — workout.

POSITIVES AND POSSIBLE PROBLEMS

My personal favourite aspect of running is that you can literally do it anywhere with nothing more than a pair of running shoes; I use it to explore when I travel, to work out whenever a gym is not accessible, and to quickly destress before any stressful meeting or media appearance. Another positive is the potential for gradual progression and never-ending fitness goals. Initially the goal of being able to

For added motivation, train with a friend or join a running group. You are less likely to skip a workout if people are waiting for you. Being social can be fun!

jog is motivating enough. Most people start by progressing up to five kilometres. Once you can run for thirty minutes or so, training for a race is a great way to stay motivated. A race goal builds in a "have to–ness"; your training has purpose and you feel like an athlete.

Another positive is that running fits with three of the four personalities. Gym bunnies, competitive athletic gym bunnies, and homebodies often gravitate toward having a training goal. Racing is rewarding. Crossing the finish line feels amazing. It makes the entire experience worthwhile. Running works for homebodies because hitting the pavement does not require a gym membership, and gym bunnies often like the flexibility inherent in running — train on the treadmill when at the gym, but ward off anxiety with the knowledge you can always run outside if the gym is not feasible that day.

The largest potential problem is injury — running is hard on the body. You can't just run. The repetitive nature stresses your joints, tendons, and ligaments, so it's essential to cross-train. Try different types of cardio workouts, strength training, core training, stretching, and self-massage with a foam roller. This is especially important when training for longer races. Endurance runners often skimp on weights and stretching because their legs are tired and training is time-consuming. I get it — I've been there. But when you're building toward a long-distance event, your body needs the strength and mobility workouts the most so that it's strong enough to handle the stress of high-intensity training. To avoid injury, time-crunched multi-taskers should hold off on race training until their schedule allows for appropriate training; it is almost impossible to safely pepper running throughout the day because you need adequate warm-up and cool-down. Even training for

I wish I could relive my first race experience. I will never forget my first half-marathon! Throughout the race I cursed my running partner, telling her I hated her for making me run. Roughly three seconds after crossing the finish line, I started smiling and said, "That was awesome! What race will we do next?" That was twelve years ago and I haven't stopped running since. My experience is not uncommon. I regularly hear almost identical "that was terrible … when can I do it again?" post-racing life moments. If you have moments while training, or during the race, where you feel like you hate running and want to give up, know that the feeling is part of the process.

Recovery
• • • • • • • • • •

Prioritize recovery. Exercise (especially high-impact activities like running) stresses the body. Give your body the ingredients it needs to recover: Get seven or more hours of sleep each night, be mindful of nutrition, and schedule time to stretch or use a foam roller, or get regular body work like massage.

a relatively short five-kilometre race requires at least two to three, twenty- to thirty-minute runs weekly. So, if you are currently truly a time-crunched multi-tasker (your workouts consist of short bouts of motion in your work clothes), then race training is not for you. Not right now anyway.

HOW TO GET STARTED

Whether you decide to just run or train for a race, make sure to progress gradually. Give your body time to adapt. At the beginning make walking intervals your friend. Space out your runs. Newbie runners should run two to three times a week on non-consecutive days. (More seasoned runners might alternate two days of running with one day of recovery.) If you're training for a race, your week should include one LSD (long slow distance) run, one speed or hill run, and one or two easier just-go runs. The distance of each run depends on your end goal. Make sure you taper in the week before your race. Decrease your training volume and intensity. Tapering allows your body to rest and helps you perform your best on race day.

For information about hill workouts and interval training, see chapter 7, Workout Plans. And if you've never ever run before, consider trying the eight-weeks-to-a-five-kilometre program outlined in the same chapter.

Half-Marathon Programs

· · · · · · · · · · ·

Most half-marathon programs call for three to five days of running per week. If you are prone to injuries, stick to three high-quality runs. Prioritize strength training and stretching. Replace the two lost running days with other forms of cardio like cycling or swimming.

Cycle, Swim, or Train for a Triathlon

PILLAR: CARDIOVASCULAR

Cycling is a fantastic method of transportation and a killer cardio and leg workout. Many people combine biking to work with triathlon training; they use their commute as part of their weekly biking mileage. Swimming is a full-body, non-impact cardio workout — ideal for cross-training or for those living with osteoarthritis.

POSITIVES AND POSSIBLE PROBLEMS

Training for a triathlon involves working three sports (cycling, swimming, and running) into your week. This — as opposed to just running — changes the load put on the body. Running is high impact; cycling and swimming are not. The sports complement each other. As with a running race goal, training for a specific triathlon race distance and date is great for staying motivated and accountable.

Competitive athletic gym bunnies are likely to gravitate toward triathlons as a training goal. Endurance cycling might also appeal to this personality — especially those who join a cycling team or group. The more advanced cyclists in the group challenge and positively push the less seasoned athletes. Homebodies might love duathlons (where you only run and bike and don't swim) since they won't have to join a gym. Swimming, unless you live at a lake or own an endless pool (if so can we be friends?), will involve a gym or community centre. Time-crunched multi-taskers often love using cycling as a method of transportation. Competitive athletic gym bunnies often find commute cycling not enough. (Personally, I find cycling in the city annoying. I hate stopping at lights and I don't find it enough of a workout. If I can't cycle on an open country road, I would much rather simply get on my indoor bike trainer and go hard for thirty to forty-five minutes.)

A large negative of cycling is the havoc it can wreak on posture. Cyclists need to prioritize stretching and posture-specific exercises, especially cyclists who also sit for work. Another possible negative is that triathlon training is time-consuming. It can be challenging to fit in three sports — and getting to the pool can be frustrating. I now do duathlons (run/bike/run) for that very reason. Again, training for a race is probably not realistic or safe for time-crunched multi-taskers, and the swimming aspect might make homebodies steer clear. Another negative is that many people find swimming in open water — especially surrounded by others — intimidating. Consider investing in a few swimming lessons to tweak your form and, if possible, practising in open water before race day.

HOW TO GET STARTED

In a triathlon you swim, bike, and run. Don't be intimidated by the three sports — there are many short races. Start with a try-a-tri (usually 350-metre swim, ten-kilometre bike, three-kilometre run) or a sprint-distance triathlon (usually 750-metre swim, twenty-kilometre bike, five-kilometre run). Make a three-month training plan and keep track of your workouts and progress. Join a triathlon club or find a few friends to go cycling in the country with on weekends. There is nothing like cycling in the country. I would consider it part of my perfect day. For a four-month sprint triathlon training plan, see chapter 7.

Fitness Classes: Pilates

PILLAR: STRENGTH AND MOBILITY

Pilates emphasizes breath regulation, mindfulness, and alignment. Mat Pilates is primarily done on the floor, focuses on training the core, and uses small apparatuses including the Pilates ring, weighted balls, the Pilates ball, and a foam roller. Pilates can also be done on machines; historically, the most popular have been the Reformer and the Cadillac Chair. One new iteration of Pilates uses the Megaformer M3, a longer, wider, and more versatile version of the Reformer.

POSITIVES AND POSSIBLE PROBLEMS

The controlled activation of the deep stabilizer muscles, especially the core, inherent to Pilates is ideal, especially if you are recovering from an injury or using it as a method of cross-training. Thus, all four personalities could benefit in some fashion if recovering from an injury or being concerned about core strength. Mat Pilates exercises don't require equipment, so homebodies typically enjoy finding sample exercises online and the time-crunched multi-tasker can easily pepper exercises into their daily life — for example at their desk. Gym and competitive bunnies can easily find classes at their local gym — virtually all gyms offer some type of Pilates. Competitive athletic gym bunnies might consider learning a few go-to exercises they do pre-sport to prime their body for motion.

The biggest potential negative — depending on your personality — is that most Pilates classes are relatively slow paced. The purpose is to connect to your body and strengthen your deep stabilizer muscles. Many people, especially competitive athletic gym bunnies, find the pace tedious. If you like the idea of Pilates, but are looking for a faster-paced, more-intense workout, classes on the Megaformer might be for you. Also note that Pilates is not a cardiovascular workout. It does not replace something like running, although it does complement higher-intensity activities.

HOW TO GET STARTED

There are two basic types of Pilates: mat and machine-based training. Mat Pilates can be an affordable option; in theory you can do it at home because all you need is your own body. That said, I absolutely suggest attending a group class or — if you can afford it — buying one or two personal sessions with a Pilates instructor before getting started. Pilates is nuanced. It can be hard to get the most out of a program online if you don't understand the underlying techniques. For example, an online program might cue you to engage your lower abdominals, but if you don't know how to do that, the instruction is useless. Once you know the basics you can easily follow online workouts. If you get bored with the basics you can purchase inexpensive small-apparatus Pilates pieces such as the band ($10), a Pilates ball ($10), or a ring ($30) to ramp up your workout.

Personally, I like going to a class. I like the variety, the accountability, and having someone watch my form. Often what I think my body is doing it actually isn't doing. If you decide to try a class, make sure to sample different instructors and studios to find the vibe you like. Make sure the instructor is certified — Stott and Body Harmonics are two popular certifications, but many are available. If you get bored of mat classes, consider attending a machine reformer class. These are particularly good if you are worried about bone health (osteoporosis) and thus want the external resistance offered by the machine. If you get bored with reformer classes you can try Lagree Pilates or springboard classes (a slightly newer variation of group Pilates done on the springboard, which is a more accessible version of the traditional Cadillac Chair created by Joseph Pilates).

Fitness Classes: Barre

PILLAR: TYPICALLY, STRENGTH AND MOBILITY
All classes include strength and mobility work. Some also include bouts of cardio.

Participants use small weighted balls or weights, the bar, a mat, resistance bands, their own body weight, and a small squishy ball to mimic the callisthenic, flexibility, and strength exercises done by dancers.

POSITIVES AND POSSIBLE PROBLEMS

Barre promotes flexibility and joint mobility, which most of us need since we tend to sit too much. When we do move, it is often in set forward-movement patterns (e.g., walking, biking, elliptical, running), which can cause stiffness and certain muscles to become stronger than others. (As a triathlete I am guilty of this — I primarily move in repetitive forward motions.) If you sit a lot or your current routine includes repetitive activities like running, barre might complement your lifestyle. As with Pilates, gym bunnies typically enjoy barre and, since most of the exercises don't require equipment, homebodies and time-crunched multi-taskers can easily find exercises online.

Barre primarily builds muscular endurance, so if you're looking to increase muscular strength or size (hypertrophy), try another class. Generally, gym bunnies and competitive athletic gym bunnies who prefer lifting heavier weights should steer clear.

HOW TO GET STARTED

First, know going in that it is a great workout and tons of fun; just don't buy into the hype that barre will give you a dancer's long and toned body. No workout — especially done once or twice a week — will get you a dancer's body if you don't have a dancer's genetics, volume of training, and diet. There are tons of different barre studios; I tend to like Barre3 the best — I have tried the brand across North America and find the instructors consistently friendly, inviting, and knowledgeable.

Fitness Classes: Spin
PILLAR: CARDIOVASCULAR

Some classes include a few minutes of strength work but not enough to (in my opinion) be considered a complete strength workout. Most end with a few minutes of mobility and stretching, but again, not enough to be considered a mobility workout.

Spin is cycling done in a group to music. The teacher guides you through varying cadences and cycling positions. You get a varied, intense, non-impact interval cardio workout.

POSITIVES AND POSSIBLE PROBLEMS

The two biggest positives of spin are improved cardiovascular and musculoskeletal strength and the extra motivation inherent in group activities. Plus, almost all gyms have spin classes of some sort, so almost anyone can try one. Gym bunnies typically enjoy a good sweaty spin class. Homebodies might enjoy spin if they are willing to invest in a home spin bike (totally possible). There are online spinning programs you can follow. Some classes are fairly competitive. Many competitive athletic gym bunnies gravitate toward this vibe and find the workout complements their other sports. Spin offers non-impact cross-training for runners, tennis players, or any athletes whose sports involve impact.

Spin is not ideal for time-crunched multitaskers. You can't pepper spin in to your day. As with any cycling, a negative of spin is the havoc it can have on your posture; in essence, cycling is sitting and we all sit way too much. Cycling is non-weight-bearing, which is ideal if you have osteoarthritis, but not ideal if you are hoping to strengthen your bones to prevent or manage osteoporosis. So, if you spin, make sure you also do weight-bearing exercises, posture-friendly strength exercises, and multi-directional activities.

HOW TO GET STARTED

If you're nervous, go with a friend — everything is better with a friend. Take the class at your own pace. The great part of spin is that although the teacher tells you to turn up your dial or increase your speed, you don't have to listen. If the class is standing you can stay seated. If the class is spinning quickly, keep your speed under control. Do what you are comfortable with. Progress as needed. Do you. Respect your body! Know that you can always leave if you need to. My suggestion is to look into the music before you go (this is often stated online). The music makes or breaks a class for me. Be prepared to try a few different classes. Find a teacher and studio you like. If your city has ClassPass use it to sample a few different studios — ClassPass can be a nice way to experiment at minimal expense.

Fitness Classes: Interval Cardio or Weight Classes

PILLARS: STRENGTH AND CARDIOVASCULAR

Most sessions end with a few stretches but not usually enough to be considered a full mobility or stretching workout.

These classes sandwich bouts of strength training between cardio, usually on a treadmill or rower. In a typical class half the participants start on the cardio machines and do prescribed intervals. The other half does weights on the floor, often using a combination of free weights, medicine balls, and bands. Then the groups switch. In some classes each group does thirty minutes of each before switching. In others you switch every ten to fifteen minutes.

POSITIVES AND POSSIBLE PROBLEMS

The largest positive is that busy individuals appreciate getting both a strength and a cardio workout in one hour — one-stop shopping. Gym bunnies often enjoy sampling different versions of these classes. Some competitive athletic gym bunnies also enjoy these classes; there is usually a vibe of competitiveness, even if the competition is only with yourself.

These workouts are not for time-crunched multi-taskers. In theory homebodies could use the principles at home (alternate between weights and cardio), but most people find the format hard to replicate. Is this class for you? That depends on your goals. They are somewhat of a compromise — you don't get a full-length cardio or a full-length weight workout. Personally, I would rather do either a full cardio workout or a full weight workout than thirty minutes of each. I don't love paying to run because I know I will run on my own. The format might work for you if you don't need a full forty-five minute to an hour strength workout or you need the outside accountability to make yourself do cardio.

HOW TO GET STARTED

Branded examples include Orangetheory, which has been in the United States for years and just opened roughly fifty gyms in Canada, and Barry's Bootcamp. Barry's Bootcamp, as one of the founders of this format, deserves a special shout-out. At Barry's you alternate sprints on Woodway treadmills (the Cadillac of treadmills) with weights. Barry's originated in New York but is currently exploding throughout North America. You absolutely don't have to go to either of these franchises. Most gyms are starting to offer their own iterations on the concept — check your local gym's schedule.

Fitness Classes: Boxing

PILLAR: TYPICALLY, STRENGTH AND MOBILITY
Primarily cardiovascular work, but many include bouts of strength and mobility work, although in my experience not enough to replace a full strength or mobility workout.

Boxing classes combine boxing with intense strength and cardiovascular moves. As my girlfriend Jenn says, boxing classes are a "sneaky way to fit in both cardio and strength; punching distracts you from a racing heart and tired arms."

POSITIVES AND POSSIBLE PROBLEMS

I personally love boxing. You leave sweaty, exhilarated, and somehow paradoxically calm;

punching can release nervous energy and pent-up frustration. I feel a similar full-body exhaustion to running, but boxing challenges the body and brain in a way that running doesn't; translating instructions — jab is one and a cross is two, et cetera — into appropriate movement is a brain workout. Gym bunnies and competitive athletic gym bunnies typically gravitate toward boxing workouts.

Now, there are negatives. Classes tend to bias strengthening the front of the body. Working the front — chest, shoulders, abdominals — over the back of the body can contribute to posture imbalances and shoulder or neck injuries. Most of us sit excessively; our bodies do not need more exercises that curl us forward. If you decide to box regularly, complement the workout with posterior-chain exercises like rows, Superwomans, chest stretches, and rotator cuff exercises such as lying external rotations.

Expense and access can also be negatives. Equipment — gloves, et cetera — can get expensive, and boxing isn't a good fit for homebodies. You need instruction, form correction, and equipment. Unless you're a real enthusiast, it is expensive to buy a punching bag for home, and without a bag — or a partner to hold pads — most people get sick of air boxing. So yes, you could do a boxercise class at home off of the internet, but I wouldn't

suggest it. Form correction is needed, and part of the absolute joy of boxing is actually punching something — either a bag or pads held by a partner. On a related note, you could pepper some air boxing into your day at work, but most time-crunched multi-taskers tend to feel silly throwing random air punches at work.

HOW TO GET STARTED

Know that although most studios say their boxing classes are appropriate for all, since punching requires the body to dissipate forces, the class presents a potential for injury — especially to the shoulders and neck. Go in knowing what is appropriate for your body, and advocate for yourself. Go early for extra instruction and ask for help when needed.

Fitness Classes: Aquafit
PILLAR: CARDIOVASCULAR

Yes, many classes do include strength work (in the water), but the strength work is not against gravity and thus is not ideal for bone health. I would suggest strength work with free weights or bands as a compliment to water activity.

Think of aquafit as aerobics in the water. Picture old-school synchronized Jane Fonda–esque aerobics, but with participants in the water trying to mimic an instructor on the deck.

POSITIVES AND POSSIBLE PROBLEMS

The main benefit of aquafit is that the water offers participants the benefits of a cardiovascular workout without wear and tear on their joints. The workout is fun, safe, and effective. It is appropriate for people with osteoarthritis or other joint complications, for anyone wanting low-impact cross-training, and for athletes recovering from injury. The water allows participants to challenge their heart and lungs without overstressing their joints. Aquafit typically also includes intervals. Intervals (bouts of high- and low-intensity training) are essential to any fitness routine. The intent behind interval training is to gradually increase your fitness so that higher-intensity work feels more normal. Gym bunnies might enjoy aquafit, depending on their age and goals.

A large possible negative is that many don't find aquafit stimulating (i.e., intense) enough. Personally, I find aquafit fun for about twenty minutes, then I'm bored. (Now this could be because I used to teach aquafit, so I often know exactly what is coming, but it could also be that many aquafit classes are boring.) It is usually not competitive enough for competitive athletic gym bunnies, too much of a time commitment for time-crunched multi-taskers, and not at home enough for homebodies.

Also, an appropriate amount of impact and stress on bones aids in prevention and management of osteoporosis. If you do aquafit regularly, great — just make sure to also walk and strength train.

Last, not everyone feels comfortable in a bathing suit, and aquafit is a big time investment. You have to budget time for transportation to and from the pool and possibly to wash and blow-dry your hair.

PILLAR BY PILLAR

I have outlined different types of fitness classes. Classes often offer a mix of all three pillars. A class might start with cardio and end with strength and mobility work — you often get a smorgasbord of a workout. Now we'll go through pillar by pillar and look at some options for your WORKOUTmix.

PILLAR NUMBER 1: STRENGTH WORKOUTS

Everyone should be doing strength and balance work. Period. Strength training is non-negotiable. It is too easy to fall into doing only cardio.

These breakdowns are of training styles and modes of training most often done at the gym solo or with a personal trainer. That said, to make it more complicated, some group classes will be described as simply a strength workout, and they include these techniques. There are innumerable training technique options including single sets, drop sets, circuit training, super-sets, and time-based training. You can also manipulate variables, such as tempo, reps, sets, weight

---

Scheduling Strength Training

When scheduling strength training workouts, be mindful that how you break up the focus on body parts — also known as your split — will depend on your goals, injury history, and schedule. Don't work the same muscle two days in a row, and aim to work each muscle group at least twice each week. Some possible splits:

- Two days a week to work out? On non-consecutive days, work your full body each day.
- Four days a week and a goal of strength and endurance? Consider two days of upper body and two days of lower body.
- Four days and a goal of hypertrophy and power? Consider chest and back one day, shoulders and legs one day, and arms and calves another day. On day four, train core and your weakest body part.

(body weight or external resistance such as dumbbells), and rest intervals.

Strength training is highly functional — it improves quality of life. It helps increase metabolism and lean muscle mass; manage mood and mitigate depression and anxiety; improve athletic performance, core strength, power, and balance; manage myriad diseases, including diabetes and high blood pressure; and decrease the risk of osteoporosis and cardiovascular disease. And let's not forget it improves body shape and composition. An inappropriate lifting program can result in injury, but you just have to be diligent at finding what fits your body and strength train intelligently. Injuries are often the result of hubris or a lack of knowledge — read the 411 of fitness again from chapter 5; make sure your splits are appropriate and that you're scheduling rest days and dividing your focus on body parts. Tailor workouts to your needs, injury history, and goals; recover appropriately; leave your ego at the door; and *always* be mindful of form.

Strength training is ideal for the gym bunny and competitive athletic gym bunny. Most athletes know that to be strong at their sport they need to be strong in the weight room. Homebodies often gravitate toward more endurance-based strength training (lighter weight, more reps) because

of space and low cost. Obviously, if you can afford a high-end home gym, the sky's your limit. Time-crunched multi-taskers need to find ways (like the piggyback method or the married technique) to fold strength and balance exercises into their life.

Training techniques and the resistance chosen will depend on your goals, level of fitness, and equipment. If you're a homebody, you might have to be creative and use only your own body weight and a TheraBand; gym bunnies have access to machines and free weights. The trick is to manipulate, when possible, the resistance, reps, and equipment to match your goals. You might have to tweak where you work out, buy new equipment, or change your goals as you become more fit. For example, if you want muscle size, you will only be able to exist as a homebody for so long before you have to buy new equipment, join a gym, or change your goals.

Some Options for Strength and Conditioning

SUPER-SETTING, TRI-SETTING, AND CIRCUIT TRAINING

With single-set (i.e., traditional) weight training, you rest between each set of an exercise; you might do three sets of ten reps with a ninety-second rest between each set. When you perform a super-set, tri-set, or circuit, you don't rest until you finish all the included exercises. In a super-set, two exercises are done back-to-back without rest. For a tri-set, three exercises. Circuits can include three or more exercises.

Individuals pressed for time love these multi-set techniques; without rest you get a more intense workout in relatively less time.

All repetition ranges and training goals work with circuit training, super-setting, and tri-setting, but each inherently works better for some goals and ranges. For example, circuit training works best for endurance training (twelve or more reps). Super-sets and tri-sets typically mesh best with a goal of eight or so reps. Traditional training and super-setting are best when lifting between your one-rep max and endurance reps of twenty. Typically, the heavier you lift, the fewer reps you will do, the more rest you need, and the fewer back-to-back sets you should do. The lighter you are lifting (the more endurance-based your training), the less rest you need and the more back-to-back exercises your body can handle.

Heavy weight, low reps, few back-to-back exercises, and ample rest exists on one side of the training continuum. Large circuits, lighter weights, and minimal rest exists on the other end.

TIME-BASED TRAINING, AMRAPS, AND MINUTES

With time-based training, the aim is not to complete a certain number of reps. Instead you work for a prescribed amount of time; perform as many reps as possible — with good form, of course — in the set time interval.

AMRAP stands for "as many rounds as possible." With AMRAP, you aim to fit in as many cycles of a circuit as possible within a set time. The faster you get through the reps, the more times you will complete the entire circuit in the time frame. Homebodies can use body-weight exercises like squats and burpees. Gym bunnies and competitive athletic gym bunnies can use anything from barbells to Bosu to cable machines.

 Try this ten-minute AMRAP. Time yourself for ten minutes. Do as many rounds as you can of ten push-ups, ten lunges each leg, twelve bent-over rows, and ten squats. Record how many rounds you get through. Work to increase the number of rounds you can complete in ten minutes.

A word of caution: Only include exercises in your AMRAP that you can do with perfect form. If you can't do squats well, try lunges. If you can't do full push-ups, try push-ups from your knees. AMRAPs are a more advanced type of training. Master the exercises first.

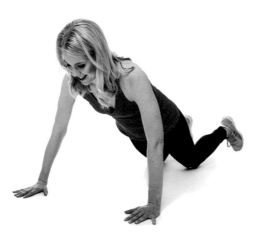

Minutes is the term for picking a series of exercises and doing each back-to-back for a minute without resting. My current favourite iteration includes six minutes of strength, three minutes of cardio, and one minute of rest. Pick four strength exercises and two core exercises. Do one minute of each exercise — aim to fit in as many good reps as possible for each exercise within each minute — followed by three minutes of intense cardio. Rest for one minute. Repeat the cycle one to three more times. I love that minutes provide an intense full-body workout in twenty to forty-five minutes, and since you are not married to any particular equipment, you can do them anywhere. You have no excuse to skip your workout! Always make your workouts convenient. You are way more likely to do them consistently if they are convenient, and consistency is key. For a sample minutes workout, see chapter 7.

OUT-OF-THE-BOX STRENGTH WORKOUTS

Out-of-the-box workouts are ideal for more advanced gym bunnies, homebodies, or competitive athletic gym bunnies who are bored and looking to spice up their routine; these workouts tend to be particularly useful for homebodies, as they don't typically have access to varied machines and thus need to manipulate the style of workout to stay motivated and challenged.

With add-on sets you alternate a base exercise with a rest exercise. Each time you do the base move, you add. The rest exercise isn't easy; it just doesn't work the same muscles as the base exercise. For example, if your base exercise is a plank (that works the core), then your rest exercise could be a squat or lunge (that works your legs). The two exercises just have to work different body parts. Confused? See the sample routine in chapter 7.

With ten-by-one-minute sets each set is broken down into ten, one-minute intervals. Within each minute, you must complete two exercises back-to-back. Done early? Relax for the remainder of the minute. If it takes you the full minute to complete both exercises then you immediately start your next interval. Feel free to experiment. Try burpees and jumping jacks. Or, if you have weights, try bent-over rows and bench presses.

When the ten minutes is up, pick two more exercises and complete another ten-minute set. If you do two sets, the workout will take twenty minutes. Feeling really brave? Add a third set.

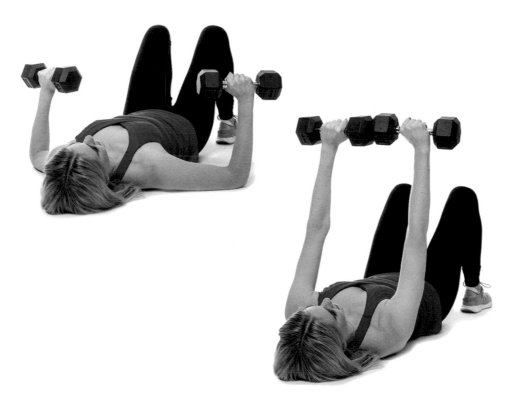

Try a sample ten-by-one-minute set.

PUSH-UPS: On your knees or toes, bend your elbows to lower your chest toward the ground. Exhale as you push yourself back up. Repeat eight times. For an extra challenge, after each push-up, try jumping your feet toward your hands and standing up. Place your hands back on the ground and jump your feet back to the starting position.

SQUATS: Stand with your feet hip distance apart. Bend at your hips, knees and ankles and sit your bum backward like you are sitting in a chair. Repeat eight times.

If you finish your eight push-ups and eight squats before the minute is up, you get to rest. If not, start again.

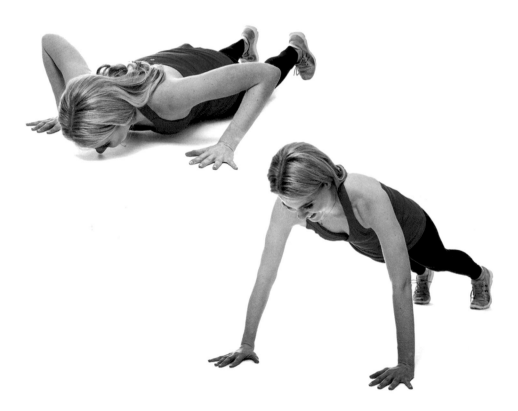

Elevens go back and forth between two exercises. The total number of repetitions should always equal eleven. For example, start with ten push-ups and one squat thrust. Then, nine push-ups and two squat thrusts. Keep decreasing the push-ups and increasing the squat thrusts by one repetition until you finish with one push-up and ten squat thrusts. Not sure what a squat thrust is? Don't worry, I got you! Start by standing with feet shoulder-width apart. Hold a dumbbell in each hand at your sides. As you squat, do a biceps curl. As you stand up, push the weights up over your head. Return the weights to their starting position and repeat. Don't have weights? Use soup cans or do squat jumps.

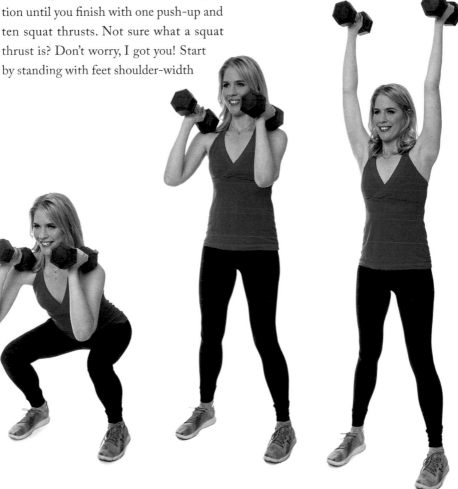

PILLAR NUMBER 2: CARDIOVASCULAR WORKOUTS

• •

Cardio workouts primarily strengthen the cardiovascular system — the heart and lungs. There are two main ways to get a cardio workout: steady-state and undulating or interval training. Both have their place. How often you do each will depend on your goals. Traditional cardio includes running, cycling, or the elliptical. More creative cardio includes dancing (maybe around your living room), roller blading, running up and down your household stairs, or jumping on a mini trampoline. Most classes — such as spin or interval strength and cardio classes — typically bias toward being interval-based cardio workouts.

Steady-State Cardio

With steady-state cardio, the goal is to maintain a relatively stable heart rate — roughly between 60 and 85 percent of your max — for most of the workout (ideally at least twenty minutes). You could also think of it as endurance cardio.

Steady-state cardio might be lovingly described as old school — intervals are currently more trendy — but there is nothing wrong with steady cardio. Steady-state may not be in vogue, but it has many positives, including strengthening the cardiovascular system, improving mood, burning calories, and strengthening connective tissues. It is also safe, accessible, and relatively unintimidating. Never let fitness trends deter you from going for an awesome bike ride or whatever makes you fitness happy.

The problem is that steady-state workouts can become boring and — relative to interval training — are less effective at burning fat and don't have the same ability to kick your fitness into the stratosphere. (That said, relative to doing nothing, a steady-state workout absolutely burns fat and improves fitness. Again, don't let the quest for perfection deter you from doing something. Just move!) I'm not saying not to do steady-state cardio. There is nothing like a steady-state run to improve my mood, and many goals, such as sport performance, require the endurance formed through steady-state workouts.

Steady-state cardio typically is less intimidating and thus fantastically habit-forming, and it's okay if, at the beginning of your health journey, steady-state cardio makes up most — if not all — of your training. Just don't make steady-state cardio your forever-and-always method of training. As you get more comfortably active, incorporate interval-style workouts. Eventually aim to include at least two interval workouts per week.

Interval Workouts

With intervals, you alternate between bouts of high- and low-intensity training. This places a high metabolic demand on the body, burns lots of calories in a short time, produces a high EPOC (which stands for "excess post-exercise oxygen consumption" and is a post-workout calorie burn), increases mitochondrial growth (mitochondria help to burn fat), and helps improve one's fitness level. I also find that keeping track of the time and shifting speeds makes my workout go faster. As a bonus, intervals are convenient — you can do them anywhere — and they keep workouts interesting. Too often people tell me they stopped training out of boredom. Of course people quit training if they find it boring — disliking something is a huge disincentive! So give intervals a try.

Think of interval training as highway versus city driving. When you come off the highway, city driving seems slow, even though before you got on the highway, city driving didn't feel slow. It was your norm. Driving faster on the highway, or working at a higher level on a cardio machine, teaches your body to understand that your normal is slow and thus helps to increase your fitness.

Don't be afraid of interval training. The myth is you have to be fit already to do intervals, but they are not just for athletes; you can do intervals without running stairs or sprinting until you puke. You alternate between bouts of higher- and lower-intensity activity, but the intensity of your interval depends on your individual fitness level. For some, the high interval will be walking quickly. For others, it might be jogging.

Competitive athletic gym bunnies will appreciate the sport-specific nature of intervals — intervals train your body to be athletic and competitive. Homebodies will appreciate the do it anywhere nature of intervals. Gym bunnies will appreciate how intervals breathe new life into stale machine workouts and add additional classes to the gym schedule (like HIIT — high-intensity interval training). Time-crunched multi-taskers will appreciate the time-efficiency of intervals, but true time-crunched multi-taskers will not be able to do most types of intervals — an intense interval workout can't be peppered into your day since it requires a good warm-up and cool-down.

Easy Pick-Ups

Warm up for five minutes. Do ten minutes at regular speed (and regular level if on a machine that has levels). Then, cycle through the following for ten minutes: alternate between thirty seconds at regular speed, twenty seconds slightly faster, and ten seconds fast. Finish with five to fifteen minutes at your regular speed and level. Cool down for five minutes.

Pyramid Intervals

VERSION A: Warm up for five minutes. Do one minute hard, one minute easy, two minutes hard, two minutes moderate, three minutes hard, three minutes moderate, four minutes hard, four minutes moderate, five minutes hard, one minute easy, and five minutes hard. Cool down for five to ten minutes.

VERSION B: Warm up for five to ten minutes. Then cycle through the following sequence: thirty seconds hard, thirty seconds recovery, sixty seconds hard, sixty seconds recovery, ninety seconds hard, ninety seconds recovery. Repeat three to six times. Cool down for five to ten minutes.

VERSION C: Do a progressive warm up lasting ten minutes — increase your intensity every two minutes over the course of the ten minutes. Then do one minute hard speed, one minute hard resistance (or hill, if you're on a treadmill), one minute moderate, two minutes hard speed, two minutes hard resistance or hill, two minutes moderate, three minutes hard, three minutes hard resistance or hill, three minutes moderate, four minutes hard, four minutes hard resistance or hill moderate, four minutes moderate. Finish with five minutes of hard work — try to push both your speed and resistance. Cool down for five to ten minutes.

Mini Pick-Ups

Warm up for five minutes. Do five minutes at regular speed. Alternate fifteen seconds hard with forty-five seconds moderate for ten minutes. Recover for two minutes, then repeat. Cool down for five to eight minutes.

Brick Workout

In a brick workout you do two different activities back-to-back without rest. As a triathlete, I do brick workouts that combine swimming and biking or biking and running. You can use any piece of equipment. For example, use the rower, then the treadmill.

BRICK PART 1: Warm up for ten minutes on any piece of equipment, then do ten minutes at the hardest intensity you can hold.

BRICK PART 2: Immediately start your second activity — do five minutes of moderate work. Then, do ten minutes at the hardest intensity you can hold. Finish with a five-minute cool-down.

Tabata

One cycle of Tabata takes four minutes. The four minutes is composed of eight sets of twenty seconds of intense work followed by ten seconds of complete rest. The wonderful

Tabata

• • • • • • • • • • •

If you are exercising to lose weight, keep in mind that Tabata, like any form of exercise, is not a magic solution. Losing weight depends on various interconnected factors including genetics, stress management, sleep patterns, exercise, and, most important, nutrition. Tabata workouts will help you burn a relatively large amount of calories in a short amount of time, but no workout will allow you to lose weight if you aren't eating properly. Concentrate on consuming a nutritionally dense diet. Limit processed foods and load up on lean proteins, healthy fats, whole grains, and lots of fresh fruits and vegetables.

thing about Tabata is that literally any exercise can be made into an interval. Here are two cardio Tabata options. Do as many as you can with good form in twenty seconds, then rest for ten. Do a total of five or six Tabata cycles and then cool down for five minutes.

BURPEES

Start standing. Bend over and place your hands on the ground in front of you. Step or jump your feet into a plank. Engage your core so your lower back doesn't arch. Jump your feet back toward your hands and stand up. Repeat. For an added challenge, jump toward the ceiling as you stand up.

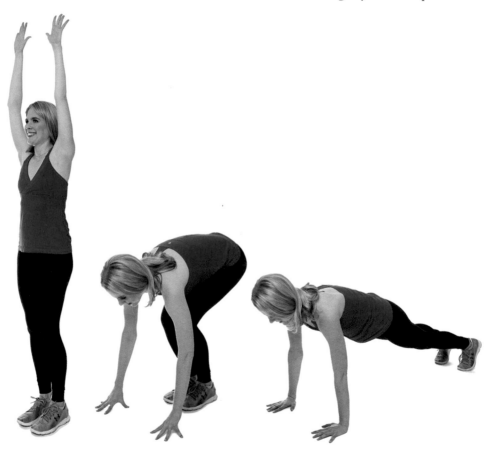

MOUNTAIN CLIMBERS

Start in a plank position. Engage your core so you're not rounding or arching your lower back. Alternate running one knee toward your chest at a time.

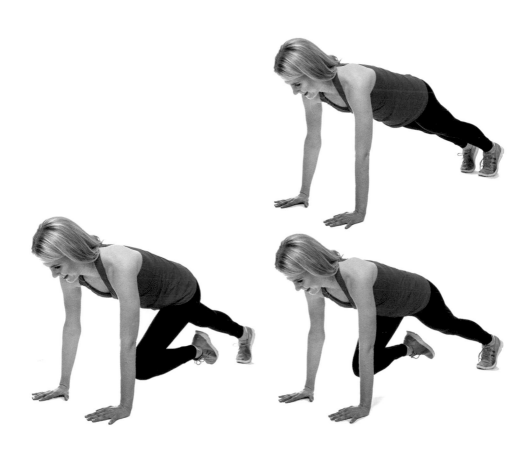

Other Cardio Options

Run up and down the stairs or do high knees, bum kicks, or lateral leaps.

Make sure Tabata workouts are appropriate for your fitness level. If you are just starting to work out, or you have a health concern like high blood pressure or diabetes, I suggest taking a more moderate approach. Try walking or light weights. Talk with your doctor to come up with an appropriate program.

FARTLEK INTERVALS

Traditional interval workouts are very detailed — based on prescribed, time-based bouts of work. Fartlek (meaning "speed play") intervals are unstructured and therefore more accessible, especially for newbies. Plus, fartlek intervals can literally be done anywhere — you have no excuse to skip your workout. Use any cardio machine, or do them while you walk, run, bike, roller blade, or even swim.

These are ideal for the time-crunched multi-tasker. They are unstructured, not necessarily overly intense, and can be done while walking or biking to work or while doing errands. Just pick a random landmark. Increase your speed until you reach it. Any landmark will do. Try a stop sign or crosswalk.

On a cardio machine, pick a random goal. Go as hard as you can until you hear the chorus in the song you are listening to or until your favourite character speaks on the TV show you are watching. If you are swimming, sprint to the end of the pool or pick a number of strokes to sprint for.

Once you hit your landmark or target, slow down and recover. Repeat for ten to thirty minutes. Finish with a cool-down and stretch.

 Bored with your workout? Need social accountability? I have the solution for you. Challenge a friend to an interval workout. Warm up for ten minutes. For the main body of the workout, take turns being the trainer and saying go. Sprint toward a destination of the trainer's choice. The trainer can make the workout as hard or as easy as they want by changing how often and how long the intervals will be.

PILLAR NUMBER 3: STRETCHING AND MOBILITY

The final pillar is mobility and stretching. I want to highlight that this pillar is not — contrary to popular practice — a when-I-have-time pillar. You have to make this pillar a priority! Try taking a class that includes mobility — yoga or Pilates — or include dynamic mobility in your warm-ups and static stretches in your cool-downs.

There are two main types of stretches: dynamic and static.

Static stretches involve holding a muscle in its lengthened position, usually for thirty seconds to two minutes. These tend to be what most people associate with "stretching." Static stretches downgrade the nervous system and cool the body down.

Save them for after your workout.

Dynamic mobility exercises warm up your body before workouts. They turn on the nervous system and prime the body for movement. They stretch muscles by moving dynamically at a joint. Put simply: dynamic mobility exercises involve motion, and static stretches are, well, static.

Dynamic stretches are ideal for competitive athletic gym bunnies before competition but can be used by all four personalities to warm up the body before exercise or even in the morning to prep the body for the day. Try the following dynamic mobility hip stretches. Dynamic and static stretches are also outlined in chapter 7.

Finding Time

Can't "find" time to stretch? Create time! Incorporate stretching into your bedtime routine, set an alarm so that you remember to do a few stretches at your desk, or stretch and use the foam roller at night as you unwind in front of the TV.

Warm Up with Dynamic Mobility Hip Stretches

I love these two hip mobilizations.

Stand with your hands against and feet away from a wall. Gently swing your left leg side to side in front of your right leg. Imagine your leg is the rope in a bell.

Next stand perpendicular to the wall, inside hand resting on the wall. Swing one leg forward and backward like a pendulum.

Keep your upper body still throughout. Repeat ten times then switch legs.

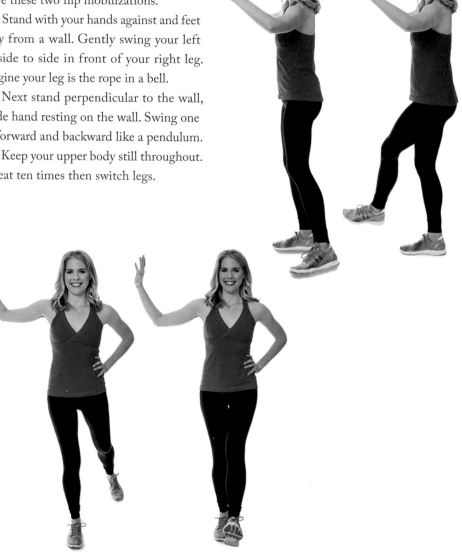

FITTING IN YOUR WORKOUTMIX

Fitting in all three pillars is often easier said than done, especially for the time-crunched multi-tasker. If you're a time-crunched multi-tasker, and you want to fit in all three pillars but can't seem to fit in a full workout, try either the married technique or the piggyback technique. Either technique could be used to fit in workouts from any of the three pillars.

The married technique involves bundling something you love — say coffee — with the healthy habit you are trying to form. For example, tell yourself you only get your coffee after you have consumed two glasses of water or have done a few stretches at your desk. The trick is to hold yourself accountable. Don't marry two things only to indulge the habit you love without doing the new healthier habit.

Gym bunnies or competitive athletic gym bunnies and homebodies can use this technique for the pillar they are having the most trouble with. For example, I am great at running and doing strength exercises, but less good at stretching. I marry TV with foam rolling and stretching.

The piggyback strategy entails pinpointing daily, non-negotiable habits you already do and turning them into a workout. It is similar to the married technique, but with this technique the non-negotiable habit you already do becomes the workout rather than simply being the trigger for you to perform a healthy habit.

This is ideal for time-crunched multi-taskers but can also be used by homebodies and gym bunnies or competitive athletic gym bunnies on days they can't fit in their regular workout — although some might not find the workout enough.

Here are some examples:

- Turn your daily dog walk into a workout using fartlek intervals. Warm up for five minutes. Pick a random landmark and speed walk, run, or sprint toward it. Walk or jog to recover. Repeat until it is time to go home. Make sure to budget for a five-minute cool down.
- Walk your child to school and then jog home.
- Instead of working or playing on your phone while waiting for your child to complete an after-school activity, bring your exercise clothes and walk

or run. If you want to watch your child practise or play, do squats and lunges on the sidelines. Or bring a mat so you can do floor work.

- Walk during conference calls or get a treadmill desk.

Get Your Steps

Track your steps on your phone or with a pedometer. Aim to increase your steps to a minimum of ten thousand per day.

- Go for a walk at lunch with a colleague.
- Get off public transit a stop early and walk to your destination.
- Park a couple of blocks from your destination.
- Walk after dinner with your partner.
- Walk to do errands.
- Constantly "forget" something in another part of your home — preferably on another floor.

NOW THAT YOU HAVE THE TOOLS, GO FORTH AND GET MOVING

You now have the tools and knowledge to create your NUTRITIONmix and WORKOUTmix. Congratulations! Hopefully you are excited to start solidifying — then actually living — your mixes.

As you start to live your mix, remember that your mix is not only unique — a little bit of this and a little bit of that or a lot of this and a little bit of that — it is also ever evolving, akin to a living organism. You don't have to be married to one workout or one version of your mix. Maybe this month you bike to work during the week and do aquafit on weekends, but during the summer you ditch aquafit in favour of swimming at the cottage. Or you train for a triathlon in the summer when you can train at your cottage, but sign up for an indoor boot camp over the winter to keep you motivated. As the seasons change, you get older, or your lived realities change so will (and should) your mix. What stays constant is that moving is always a non-negotiable; how you move is up for negotiation.

If living your mix sounds intimidating — if you're still not sure how to actually implement the information — know that some trepidation is normal. Adopting a healthier lifestyle is a big change, and I have given you a lot of information. Take a deep breath — feeling slightly overwhelmed is completely appropriate at this point in your process. Chapters 8 and 9 will help you develop your MINDSETmix — your mindset and motivation.

Your MINDSETmix will allow you to connect the dots between the desire to trend positive and the act of actually trending positive. One thing to keep in mind as you work to create your final mix is, don't get caught in the weeds. Too much analysis is paralysis. The techniques in chapters 8 and 9 will be helpful, but in the end you have to start. Anne Lamott offers the excellent advice during her TED talk that to be a good writer you need "bum in the seat time" — all writers have unusable first drafts, but good writers get over the fear of starting and reworking and "just write." As a writer I can tell you that is true. My first drafts always suck, but then I work on them — I tweak and tweak — and they get better. The same is true for being fit. Fit people have lots of bum in the workout seat time; they put their fear of sucking to the side, and they move — they just fit. Fit people embrace that their first draft of fitness will not be the final draft, and that is okay. The first draft is needed for the second and the third draft to exist. As with writing, you need to start being active so you have something to work with.

Your future self will always be happier if you move, eat well, sleep, and generally make productive and healthy decisions. You can tweak your mixes as you go, but if you don't start, you have nothing to tweak.

Don't let the quest for perfection be the enemy of getting shit done.

Change your narrative. Decide who you want to be — and be it!

CHAPTER 7

Workout Plans

In chapters 5 and 6 I explained the three pillars required for every WORKOUTmix — strength, cardiovascular, and stretching and mobility — and broke down the pros and cons of various exercise classes, training principles, and workout styles. After finishing chapter 6 you should have the tools and information needed to formulate your balanced and appropriate individualized WORKOUTmix.

The fly in the ointment? If you are not a trainer, workout theory can feel somewhat nebulous; I get that telling you to train for a five-kilometre race or try pyramid sets is not as useful as step-by-step instructions breaking down how to train for the race or giving you clear examples of what exercises to use in the pyramid set.

To combat this pesky fly, this chapter details a few concrete examples of the workouts suggested in chapters 5 and 6: five-kilometre running and triathlon training plans, detailed instructions on how to do add-on sets, minutes, and pyramid sets, and examples of pre- and post-workout stretches and mobility exercises.

By now you know to incorporate whichever examples fit into your mix.

This is by no means a comprehensive list; these examples are just the tip of the workout iceberg. There are so many fun workouts, exercises, modes of training, and fitness classes. Experiment. Try different workouts. The world is your fitness oyster — be curious!

EIGHT WEEKS TO FIVE KILOMETRES

PILLAR: CARDIOVASCULAR

Not a runner but always dreamed of being one? Need an effective, efficient, and accessible do anywhere cardiovascular workout? Thrive on time-sensitive or competitive goals? If so, training for a five-kilometre race might be for you. This program is ideal for the newbie runner. I've also included sample hill and interval workouts for when you are more experienced and ready to ramp up your fitness.

The Plan

Do all workouts three times a week on non-consecutive days.

For the first five weeks, do a five-minute power walk to warm up. Starting in week six, warm up by jogging at a speed you consider easy for five minutes. Power walk for five minutes to cool down throughout the program.

At the end of each week, do a body check. Ask yourself, Do I have any negative joint or muscle aches or pains? Muscle tiredness (or what I call positive pain) is okay, but if you have joint irritation that lasts more than forty-eight hours after a run, rest or cross-train. Try water running or Pilates. Left untreated, minor aches and pains can become full-blown acute injuries or chronic conditions. Once the negative pain has dissipated, repeat that same training week again. Progress to the next week of the program when you have no negative pain.

- **WEEK ONE:** Alternate three minutes of jogging with two minutes of walking six times.

- **WEEK TWO:** Alternate three minutes of jogging with one minute of walking six times.

- **WEEK THREE:** This week you get to try a pyramid workout. Jog for three minutes, walk for one, jog for four minutes, walk for one, jog for five minutes, walk for two, jog for four minutes, walk for one, jog for three minutes, walk for one.

- **WEEK FOUR:** Alternate five minutes of jogging with one minute of walking six times.

- **WEEK FIVE**: Congratulations! You have earned a down week; purposely don't increase the intensity of your workouts this week to ensure your body is recovering properly. Do the workout from week four again, but on two days rather than three. Cross-train and stretch.

- **WEEK SIX**: Jog for five minutes, walk for one, jog for seven minutes, walk for one, jog for eight minutes, walk for one. Jog for seven minutes, walk for one, jog for five minutes, walk for one.

- **WEEK SEVEN**: This week is simple. Jog for nine minutes and walk for one minute three times.

- **WEEK EIGHT**: Alternate between jogging for ten minutes and walking for one minute for thirty-three minutes total.

You are now jogging for a total of thirty minutes, which means you are covering roughly five kilometres every time you train. Your next goal is to either increase the time you run without a walk break or to work on speed with intervals. Try alternating fifteen minutes of jogging with one minute of walking. Or try the following interval workout: Jog for ten minutes, walk for one. Then alternate fifteen seconds of faster running with forty-five seconds of jogging at your regular speed for ten minutes. Walk for one minute. Finish by jogging at your regular speed for ten minutes.

SAMPLE PLAN: HILL WORKOUT

Hill workouts of varying lengths, splits, and speeds exist, but this is one of my favourites: Locate a hill that is approximately one kilometre away. Run to the hill then up it quickly. Walk back down. Repeat. Start with three hill repeats and work up to six to eight. Finish by jogging back to your starting location.

SAMPLE PLAN: INTERVAL WORKOUT

Interval (or sprint) workout options are endless. Here's one of my favourites: First, run for one to two kilometres to warm up. Then do two to four sets of half a kilometre at ten to forty seconds faster than your ideal ten-kilometre race speed. Walk or jog for one to two minutes between intervals. Run one to two kilometres to cool down.

FOUR-MONTH SPRINT TRIATHLON TRAINING PLAN

PILLAR: CARDIOVASCULAR

Thrive on competition or time-sensitive goals? Enjoy variety? Used to swim or run in high school or college and miss the athleticism? Enjoy being outdoors? If so, training for a triathlon might be for you. This is ideal for a newbie triathlete.

Divide your training into four, one-month training blocks.

- **MONTH ONE:** Do each sport once a week. Start with a twenty-minute swim, thirty-minute bike, and thirty-minute run. Progressively increase the duration of your workouts. By the end of the month, you should be swimming for forty minutes, biking for an hour, and running for forty-five minutes.

- **MONTH TWO:** Continue to increase the duration of your ride until you can bike continuously for an hour and a half. Add in a fourth workout per week and do whichever is your weakest of the three sports.

- **MONTH THREE:** Swim, bike, and run once per week for thirty to forty-five minutes each. In addition, do one brick workout every week. Brick workouts involve doing two sports back-to-back without resting. Once a week, bike for one to one and a half hours, then without resting, run for ten to thirty minutes.

- **FINAL MONTH:** Continue your workout plan from month three, but during a few of your shorter mid-week workouts, after you warm-up, alternate one minute of hard work with two minutes of moderate work. Do five to eight sets of these intervals.

Also aim to do two full-body strength workouts weekly. Stretch after every workout. Whenever weather permits, run, bike, and swim outside.

One week before the race, decrease the amount you are training so you are rested and ready to race.

MINUTES WORKOUT

. . . .

PILLAR: STRENGTH

Not a workout newbie but need a fast and efficient do anywhere workout? Don't have access to fancy gym equipment? Strapped for time? Travelling and want to work out in your hotel room? Want an intense workout in the comfort of your living room? If so, then this workout might be for you.

Minutes are generally not for newbie exercisers. Master the basic moves and aim for a certain number of repetitions before moving to time-based training. I suggest this for the more seasoned homebody or gym bunny who wants an intense workout but needs to get in and out of the gym quickly.

What are minutes? Minutes are a type of time-based training. In time-based training, instead of aiming to complete a certain number of reps, you aim to complete as many reps as possible (with good form) in a set time. Time-based training is effective, but more important, it is both efficient and convenient; since you are not married to any particular pieces of equipment, you can do it anywhere. You have no excuse to skip your workout! I always tell my clients that the more convenient your workout is, the better. You are much more likely to do the workout *consistently* if it is *convenient*. When it comes to achieving any health and wellness goal, consistency is key.

With minutes you do a minute of each exercise. You could do ten different exercises each for a minute and repeat the cycle one to three times. Or 5 different exercises each for 1 minute repeating the cycle one to six times. Or even twenty different exercises each for a minute. You could even do a bout of cardio between your set of minutes. There are no set rules, except within each minute you do as many reps of one exercise as you can with good form.

Sample Plan

In this version of minutes do a chest exercise (in this example, the pec-deck plank), a minute of a type of squat, a minute of an upper-back exercise (here, bent-over rows), a minute of a type of lunge, and two minutes of core followed by three minutes of cardio. Warm up for five minutes.

MINUTE 1. Pec-deck plank: Grab two towels (or gliders). If you are working out on carpet, use paper plates. Start in a plank position on your forearms and toes with one towel, glider, or plate under each forearm. This is a very challenging exercise; I suggest starting on your knees. Maintain your plank as you slide your forearms out to the side. Maintain a ninety-degree angle at your elbows. Use your chest to pull your arms back in. The movement should resemble the motion used on the pec-deck machine at the gym. If you can maintain good form from your knees, try the exercise from your toes.

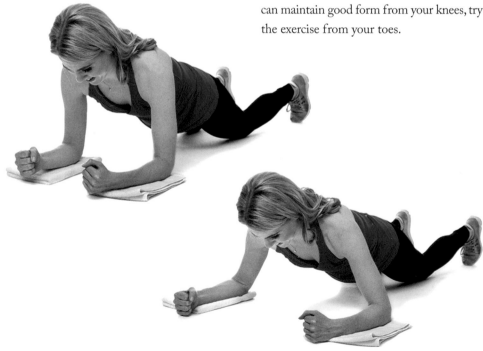

MINUTE 2. Some version of the squat: Use your own body weight, dumbbells, or a barbell. For an extra challenge, do squats standing on a Bosu.

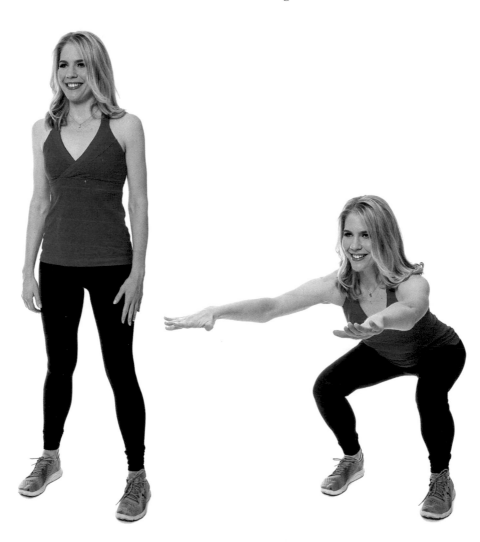

MINUTE 3. Rows: Either bent-over rows using dumbbells or standing rows using bands.

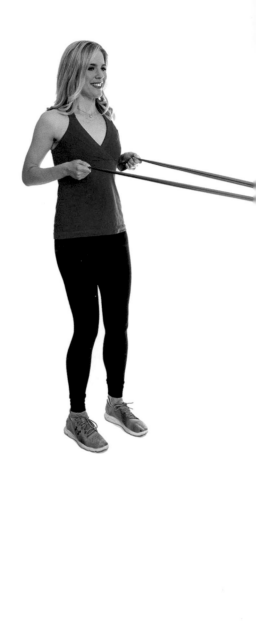

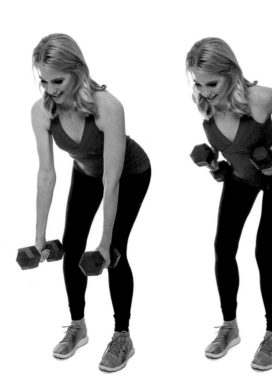

MINUTE 4. Lunges: Try walking, stationary, or Bosu lunges. For variety try a glider burnout lunge: Start standing with your right toes on a towel, glider, or paper plate. Bend your left knee and slide your right leg behind you into a low lunge. Hold. Without standing up, slide your right knee in and out. Keep your left leg still. Don't bounce. Try thirty seconds on each leg. If you really want to challenge yourself, add an extra minute to the program and try a minute on each leg.

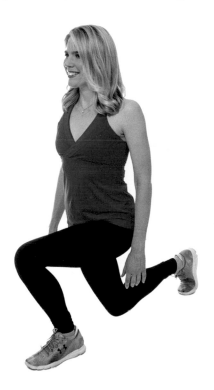

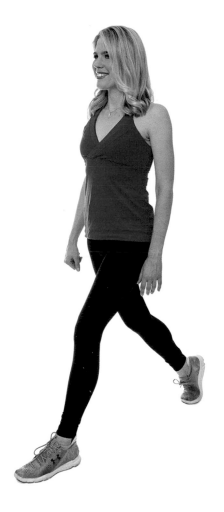

MINUTES 5 AND 6. Two core exercises: Try any variation of the V sit (see top right), front plank, or side plank. If you are sick of basic planks, try plank and hooks (see bottom left and right): Grab two towels, gliders, or paper plates. Start in a plank position on your forearms and knees or toes with one towel, glider, or plate under each forearm. Keep your pelvis stable as you slide your right arm along the floor in an arc around your left arm, like you are trying to reproduce a boxer's jab. Move your right arm for thirty seconds. Then do thirty seconds with the left.

Finish with three minutes of cardio intervals on any cardio machine. If you're not at the gym, run up and down your stairs, do burpees or high knees, skip rope, or dance around. Repeat two or three more times and cool down and stretch.

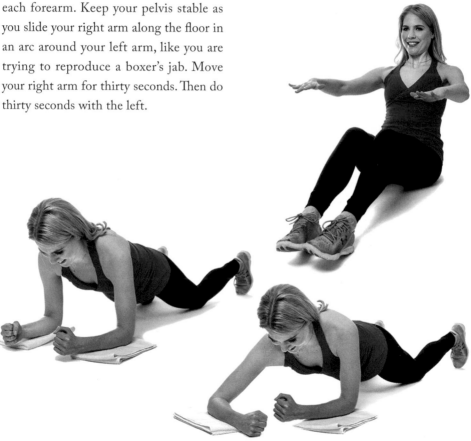

ADD-ON ROUTINE

PILLAR: STRENGTH

Not a gym rat? Enjoy training at home or in a hotel room when you travel? No access to fancy equipment? Not a workout newbie but need a fast and efficient do-anywhere workout? Strapped for time? Then this workout might be for you. I suggest this for the more seasoned homebody or gym bunny who is craving variety (boredom is the kiss of workout death) or wants an intense workout but needs to get in and out of the gym quickly.

With add-on sets you pick a base exercise and a rest exercise. The rest exercise isn't easy, it just doesn't work the same muscles as the base exercise. So, if the base exercise is a core exercise, the rest should be legs. If the base exercise is legs, make the rest an upper body or core exercise. To do the workout you simply alternate the base exercise with the rest exercise. Each time you do the base move, you add on an exercise.

In the example here, I have used a front plank as my base exercise (other options include a side plank or a V hold) and a squat hold as my rest exercise (other options include a plié hold or cardio exercises such as jumping jacks or high knees).

Add-on sets are not for newbie exercisers. Why not? You need to master the base move — with perfect form — before adding anything on. So, for example, before trying the below workout, master the basic plank first.

Basic plank: Balance on your hands and toes. Your shoulders, hips, and feet should form a straight line. Your bum should not be up in the air. Your lower back should not be arched. If I put a foam roller lengthwise along your back, the roller should touch the back of your skull, your upper back, and your sacrum (back of your pelvis).

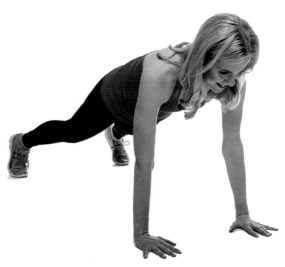

There should be a small space between the roll and both your lower back and your cervical spine. Keep your core engaged the entire time; pull your belly button toward your spine and your lower abdominals wide to your hip bones like you are pulling taffy.

SAMPLE PLAN: CORE EXTRAVAGANZA

Start standing. Bend over. Place your hands on the ground in front of you. Walk your hands forward until your body forms a plank. Hold for five seconds. This is your base exercise.

Now, walk your hands backward and, without standing all the way up, hold a squat. Keep your chest out, back flat, core engaged, knees in line with your middle toes, and lower back neutral. This is your rest exercise. After each add-on, hold a squat for five seconds. Then walk forward into your plank and start the sequence again.

ADD-ON 1. Walk-outs: After holding the basic plank for five seconds, add on walk-outs. In a plank position walk your right hand in front of you, then your left. To finish, place your right hand back to its starting position underneath you, then your left. Repeat starting with your left hand.

Walk your hands backward. Hold your low squat for five seconds.

ADD-ON 2. Shoulder taps: Walk forward into a plank. Hold for five seconds. Do one walk-out starting with each hand. Then add on shoulder taps. Keep your hips stable as you touch your right hand to your left shoulder and then your left hand to your right shoulder.

Walk your hands backward. Hold your low squat for five seconds.

ADD-ON 3. Leg extensions: Repeat the above sequence. Then, holding your plank — core engaged and pelvis stable — engage your right bum muscle to lift your right leg off the floor. Hold for five seconds and repeat with your left leg.

Walk your hands backward. Hold your low squat for five seconds.

ADD-ON 4. Leg abductions: Repeat the sequence. Then do one leg abduction with each leg. Holding your plank — core engaged and pelvis stable — engage your right bum muscle to lift your right leg off the floor and out to the side (see page 153). Hold for five seconds then repeat with your left leg.

Walk your hands backward. Hold your low squat for five seconds.

ADD-ON 5. Knee tucks: This is your final add-on. Repeat the entire sequence (while smiling, if you can), then do one knee tuck with each leg. Hold your plank as you bring one knee into your chest. Count to five. Repeat with the other leg.

Walk your hands backward. Hold your low squat for five seconds.

Jump on a cardio machine and do five minutes of intervals — fifteen seconds hard and forty-five seconds regular. Then, repeat the sequence again.

Once you can do the full routine with perfect form, hold weights when you squat and try doing two repetitions of each add-on. Progress until you can do three repetitions of each exercise.

- ten squats
- thirty seconds plank
- ten squats and ten squat pulses (hold low and pulse up and down slightly)
- thirty seconds plank
- ten squats, ten squat pulses, and thirty seconds isometric squat hold (hold at bottom range of motion for thirty seconds)
- thirty seconds plank
- ten squats, ten squat pulses, thirty seconds isometric squat hold, and thirty squat jumps (as you stand up from your squat swing your arms and propel yourself up into the air but land softly)

SAMPLE PLAN: ADD-ON LOWER-BODY BLASTER

In this version you use squats as your basic exercise and planks as your rest. If you are relatively new to training (six months or less) do body weight squats. If you are a master at squats, hold dumbbells when doing all of the squats *except* for the jumping squats.

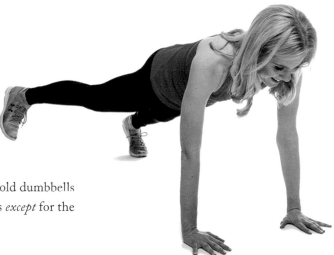

PYRAMID SET

PILLAR: STRENGTH

Pyramid sets are fantastic for gym bunnies, competitive athletic gym bunnies, or homebodies who have been training for more than six months and are looking to add variety to their routine. Why? The body is highly adaptive; if you always do the same workout it will stop responding. Eventually you will hit a fitness plateau. And who wants to repeat the same routine day in and day out?

In a pyramid set, the number of repetitions you do increases or decreases throughout the workout. The weight you use usually changes in an inverse relationship to the repetitions you are doing. What that means is, usually the fewer the repetitions, the higher the weight.

Sample Plan: Pyramid Set of Squats

Warm up with a light weight for fifteen repetitions, then do ten reps, eight reps, and six reps, increasing the weight each time.

To really get wild and crazy, super-set two exercises together within your pyramid workout. A super-set is when you do two exercises back-to-back with no rest in between. To do a super-set pyramid you need to first pick two exercises. Any two will do, but I like picking one lower-body and one-upper body exercise.

For example, you could super-set lunges and bent-over rows. Do fifteen repetitions of each back-to-back using a light weight. Rest for sixty seconds.

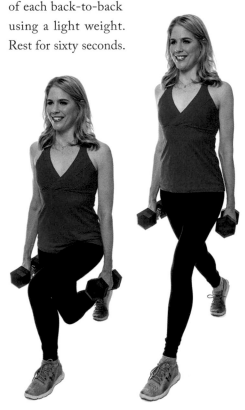

Then do ten reps of each back-to-back with a medium weight. Rest for sixty seconds. Finish with six reps of each exercise back-to-back with a heavy weight.

The repetitions don't always have to pyramid down. You can increase the repetitions as you go. I find this type of pyramid works well as a cardio warm-up.

BAND WORKOUT

PILLAR: STRENGTH

The band is ideal for the newbie lifter, the homebody, and anyone who needs to stay fit as they travel. Why? The resistance band is light and inexpensive (roughly $10). Or, invest in a doorframe attachment (under $10) to create a makeshift cable machine. The attachment is a small piece of fabric that has a ball at one end and a loop at the other. You anchor the ball into the closed door and thread the band through the loop. This allows you to replicate any exercise traditionally performed on a cable machine — wood chops, rows, triceps press downs, et cetera.

Sample Plan: Full-Body Band Workout

Warm-up (five minutes): Dance around your room or choose five different cardio moves — high knees, bum kicks, and so on. Do each for one minute.

Main circuit (repeat two to three times): Rows with doorframe attachment: squats and rows, twelve to fifteen reps.

Loop the band through the attachment. The attachment should be at roughly chest height. Hold one end of the band in each hand. Stand with your feet hip-distance apart. Bend at your hips, knees, and ankles and sit your bum backward like you are sitting in a chair. Keep your arms straight as you squat. As you stand up, use your upper back to pull your elbows backward. Imagine cracking a walnut between your shoulder blades. Slowly release.

Don't have a doorframe attachment? Try seated V hold and rows, twelve to fifteen reps.

Sit on your bum with the band hooked around your feet. Hold one end of the band in each hand. Lean back ten degrees and hold the lean throughout the motion. Engage your core to stay stable. Use your upper back to row your elbows backward. Crack the walnut between your shoulder blades. Slowly release.

Lunge and lateral raises/lunge and front raises, twelve to fifteen reps per side: Start standing with your right leg forward, foot in the middle of the band. Hold one end of the band in each hand, arms straight by your sides. As you lunge down bring your arms up to shoulder height — keep them straight. Lower your arms as you stand up (lateral raise).

To lunge, bend both knees so your body moves toward the floor. Use the bum muscle of the front leg to stand back up. When you do the exercise on your left leg, straighten your arms forward to chest height (front raise).

Overhead triceps extension, twelve to fifteen reps per side: Stand and hold one end of the band in your right hand. Reach your left hand behind your body and anchor the band. The closer your hands are together, the harder the exercise will be. Keep your right upper arm into your right ear as you straighten the arm. Slowly release.

Do one to three minutes of any cardio (burpees, high knees, jumping jacks, et cetera).

Rest for a minute. Have some water. Repeat the entire circuit.

DYNAMIC STRETCHES

• •

PILLAR: STRETCHING AND MOBILITY

Dynamic mobility exercises are a great addition to any warm-up, especially for those who feel stiff and immobile. As noted in chapter 6, dynamic mobility exercises (versus static stretches) are ideal for a warm-up because they turn on the nervous system and prime the body for movement. Dynamic mobility exercises are exercises that stretch muscles by moving dynamically at a joint.

Sample Plan:
Full-Lower Body Primer

PART 1. Step your right leg forward so you are stretching your left calf — right knee bent, left leg straight, left heel pressing down into the ground behind you. Hold for three seconds.

PART 2. Then bring your left knee up into your chest. Balance on your right leg for three seconds hugging your left knee into you.

PART 3. Repeat on the other leg. Step the left leg forward so that you stretch your right calf. Make sure to keep both feet facing forward, your back leg straight, and your front knee bent.

PART 4. Step your right leg forward into a lunge stretch. Tuck your pelvis slightly so you bring your right hip bones toward your ribs. Reach your right arm up toward the ceiling. Don't hold for any length of time — simply move through the motion.

PART 5. Repeat by stepping your left leg forward into a lunge stretch.

Move through the entire sequence two or three times.

STATIC STRETCHING

• •

PILLAR: STRETCHING AND MOBILITY

Static stretches are a vital part of any cool-down, but particularly important for the *hypo*mobile folks among us (the really stiff folks). Not everyone is tight, some of us are *hyper*mobile — our joints are too mobile. If you are hypermobile keep your stretches at a three out of ten intensity. Use static stretching to cool down your nervous system and return your body to homeostasis post workout rather than aiming to increase your mobility. (Meaning, don't push it.)

Sample Plan

A few of my favourite post workout stretches are the 90/90, the kneeling hip-flexor stretch, the standing calf stretch, and the foam roller upper-back release.

Hold each stretch for a minimum of thirty seconds. Never stretch so far that you experience pain.

1. Start sitting on the floor with your legs at 90/90 — one in front bent at ninety degrees across your body and the other behind at ninety degrees. Keep your chest out and your back flat. Hinge over your front thigh.

2. To do a keeling lunge hip-flexor stretch, start kneeling on your right knee with your left foot on the floor in front of you. Keep both hips forward. Feel the stretch up the front of your right thigh. Reach your right arm up. Hold for thirty seconds before switching legs.

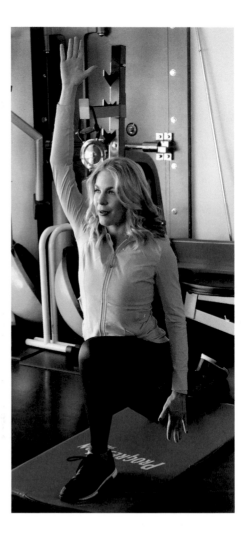

3. For a standing calf stretch, stand on a step with the ball of your right foot on the edge. Let your right heel fall toward the ground. Hold for thirty seconds before switching legs.

4. I also love using the foam roller to massage out tight muscles. If you sit at a desk, the upper-back foam roller exercise, described on page 160, is a must.

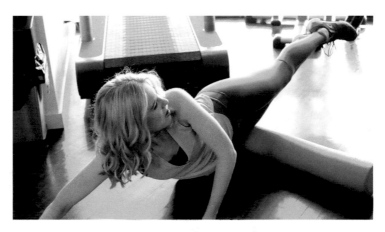

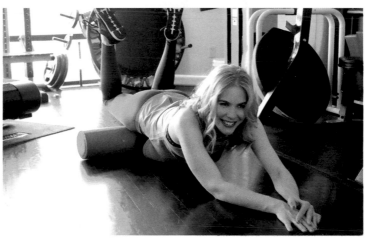

Sample Plan: Foam Roller

UPPER-BACK RELIEF: (Do you sit at a desk? If so, this is for you.) Start on the floor with your bum on the ground and the roller under your upper back, perpendicular to your body, head resting in your hands. Lift your hips up. Roll your body forward and backward so the roller moves up and down your back. Keep your core engaged.

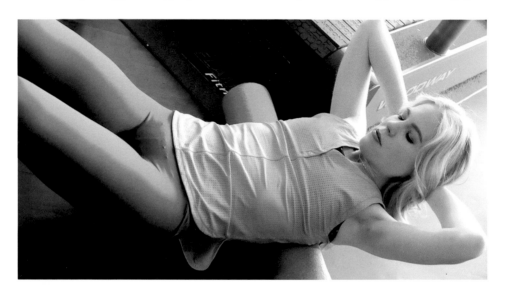

MAKE THE WORKOUTS YOUR OWN

Remember, try only the workouts that fit your mix. Do you.

Try something and don't love it? No problem, research others. One of the most important ideas in *Your Fittest Future Self* is that all experiences are simply data. If you don't love a workout — great. You now know that is not for you. If you try something and love it — fantastic — do that workout until it is boring.

Remember, the only non-negotiable is that you move. How you move is up to you!

CHAPTER 8

Setting Up for Your MINDSETmix

Your mindset is your inner dialogue — your North Star, your philosophy, your inner well of resilience and determination — built on objective scientific health facts and the motivation and mindfulness techniques that best serve you.

By now you have the information needed to create your WORKOUTmix and NUTRITIONmix. The problem is, knowing *what to do* is only half the battle — the easy half.

As I mentioned in chapter 2, Dr. Fordyce, a seminal thinker in cognitive behavioural theory and movement re-education, is credited with having first said, "Education is to behavior change as spaghetti is to brick." Action is not the automatic child of education; having knowledge does not inherently imbue us with the ability or determination to act.

Action is the result of purposeful research, self-reflection, integration of reflection on past and present behaviour, preparation, goals, hope, self-efficacy, identity and value alignment, grit, an internal locus of control, and an ability to persevere and put one foot — continually — in front of the other.

In short, living your NUTRITIONmix and WORKOUTmix — rather than just talking about them — requires the development of an individualized, flexible — resilient — mindset.

Chapters 8 and 9 break down how to create this mindset. Chapter 9 will take you through various strategies to overhaul your mindset, and to increase both motivation and mindfulness. I breakdown the pros and cons of each strategy so that you can create the recipe that works for you. This chapter gives you the skills needed to parse out appropriate information. I start with a brief explanation of *mindset* — so you know why the creation of this mix is important. Then I outline how to consciously shift your awareness, why doing you is critical, and the seven questions critical for mix-making success.

THE 411 ON MINDSET

• •

Your mindset is an inner dialogue — your philosophy of life and inner well of resilience and determination — built on objective scientific health facts and the motivation and mindfulness techniques that best serve you. It is the unique mix of motivation strategies and mindfulness techniques that respects who you are, who you want to be, and how best to mind the gap in between.

Mindset, motivation, and mindfulness are inextricably linked; the three flow from and into one another — one does not exist without the other. Your mindset reflects what you — consciously and unconsciously — pay attention to, both the stimuli and the response. Your response either alters or reinforces your mindset.

Awareness brings choice. A mindset shift requires an awareness shift. Mindfulness is required to know what the focus of your new awareness should be — for example, to know you need more vegetables, you first need to know how many vegetables you are consuming. Then, to change actions, motivation is required. See how motivation and mindfulness are inextricably linked to mindset? You can't create a new mindset if you are not aware of your actions, and you can't alter motivational patterns and thoughts when unaware of current actions and feelings. To create your fitter future self, you need to first become aware of how you react and what you react to. Only then can you work to form new habits, thoughts, actions, and patterns.

Mindfulness and understanding can — ideally — provide motivational fodder. For example, once you are aware of being bored with your current workout, that you feel crappy after eating dairy, that you are energized after running, or that you are motivated by training with a partner, you can use this awareness to foster motivation. Try a new workout, drink almond milk, book runs before key meetings to create energy, and set workout dates with friends.

Think of your mindset — your consciousness and subjective reality — as a strobe light in the forest; it illuminates only the objects within the parameters of the strobe. Further away, objects are less clear. Only when you are conscious of something — when the strobe is over that part of your life — are objects seen. To change your consciousness, change the position of the strobe.

Your NUTRITIONmix, WORKOUTmix, and MINDSETmix are all part of your overall health — and health is a process. The goal is simply for your sense of well-being and health to trend positive. As part of this trending positive process — notice the emphasis on process — think of your health in its totality. Don't fall into the all-too-common mindset of "I am licensed to make this unhealthy choice because I made this other healthy

Think Big Picture

· · · · · · · · · · ·

As you create your MINDSETmix, aim to make health choices that complement one another, not myopic one-off decisions. To do this, visualize your health in its totality; conceptualize all the pieces — your values, genetics, lifestyle, goals, nutrition and fitness choices, fitness and change personalities, et cetera — as pieces of a puzzle that fit together. Aim for choices that trend your health process forward in its totality.

choice." Don't try to game the system; don't work out so that you can eat cake or drink three glasses of wine. I am not saying never eat cake. Remember my love it rule: Go ahead and have a small portion of something you love, but have it because you have decided the experience is worthwhile, not because you think your workout has given you carte blanche to eat anything.

RECOGNIZING YOURSELF TO FIND YOUR MINDSETMIX

• •

As you create your MINDSETmix, consider these umbrella suggestions and never forget to do you.

Rule bound individuals thrive on strict lines to work within — well-established non-negotiables. Choice is confusing and overwhelming. If this is you, as you read through the motivation, mindset, and mindfulness techniques, consider how the strategies could be formed into well-defined rules or goals. Take mindset strategy 1, sleep: Consider establishing clear quantity rather than quality goals. My sleep patterns drastically improved after deciding nothing less than six and a half hours is acceptable. I am very rule bound. A benefit of being rule bound? Each time you successfully follow your rule, you get a clear little win, and small successes often positively spiral into further wins.

Go with the flow individuals need flexibility — too many rules are suffocating. This personality thrives on a fluid feeling to their day. They can adopt (or not) health habits depending on the situation and mood. If this is you, consider how you would make each technique flexible enough that you don't feel penned in but regular enough that it will make a difference.

Individuals who believe small changes add up are motivated by perseverance, not overnight success. These individuals truly believe that health is an aggregate of smaller choices. Like drops in a bucket, over time the health bucket will overflow. If this is you, as you read through the motivation, mindset, and mindfulness techniques, consider which routines would best suit you — how can you make a small habit routine enough that it eventually fills your bucket, but small enough that it still feels manageable? If you're making small changes, they have to be frequent. For example, if you drink multiple cups of coffee per day, the relatively minor act of eliminating the sugar will eventually make a big difference. If you drink one coffee per day, the small act might not accumulate in a noticeable way. It's still a good idea to cut sugar from your coffee — just match your expectations to the act and consider cutting sugar from elsewhere as well.

If big changes make you feel in control, a large jolt — a fast initial result — is motivating. Small changes feel too incremental. As you read through the techniques, consider which strategies are large enough to make you feel like you are doing something but realistic enough to be enforceable. Big changes can be motivating, but not if they are more akin to wishes; if you wish something and don't follow through, you automatically feel beaten down. You might consider the 180 daily pyramid method for change (see chapter 2).

If you make decisions because it's right (scientifically, morally just, et cetera), feel free to research my suggestions; find facts to corroborate — or counter — my recommendations. Decide for yourself if it's right. If the suggestion doesn't mesh with your values, don't adopt it. For example, to motivate yourself to get more sleep, research the science behind sleep deprivation. Then, use the facts as part of your internal dialogue when you want to stay up late and watch unnecessary TV.

If you are intrinsically motivated, connect the suggestion to your own experiences and emotions. Ask yourself if the habit would make you feel proud, happy, or joyful. Would you feel a sense of accomplishment? Connect to positive past experiences. Follow the suggestions you know will mesh with your internal barometer. If you don't know, try the techniques and journal your responses. For example, if you're thinking of using sleep as a motivational tool, journal how you feel on days you do and don't sleep. Note your energy and ability to say no to sugar and yes to working out. If you always have higher energy and resilience on days you sleep, remind yourself of that on nights you don't want to prioritize sleep. Or on days you want to make an unhealthy choice, say, "Self, this is my lack of sleep talking. I am *not* my unhealthy thought. Resist!"

As you read through the strategies, keep your exercise personalities at the forefront of your analysis — are you a gym bunny, homebody, competitive athletic gym bunny, or time-crunched multi-tasker? Be aware of your current personality and, if applicable, the personality you might be in the future. Remember to make goals not wishes. Be realistic. If your present lifestyle makes fun fitness classes a non-starter but working out at home is realistic, don't waste time wishing you could do a class. Go online and buy a home version. Or make a mental note that in a few months, when you are less busy, a class might be a great way to feel motivated. Work with what you have. Stay in your own fitness lane. Find solutions not excuses. Match your workout personality to your life circumstances, values, and goals.

SEVEN QUESTIONS TO HELP FIND YOUR MINDSETMIX

· ·

As you find your mix, ask yourself the following questions. The answers will offer valuable insight regarding your triggers, your thought loops, and your values and philosophies — all information that is vital when forming a MINDSETmix. At times when you fall, revisit the questions to help get back on the horse as a more informed rider.

1. **WHAT IS UPSTREAM OF THIS?** Our current thoughts and actions are typically inspired by previous thoughts and actions. Instead of simply addressing the symptom (current action or belief), work to understand the cause — the thought or action that got you to this place and time. What set the stage for the now? Analyze what thoughts and actions are upstream of whatever habits or actions you are attempting to change. Do you eat because of toxic thoughts? Are your hunger pangs connected to boredom? Are you depressed? Pick the mindset or motivation trick that addresses whatever is upstream.

2. **AM I EQUIPPED TO HANDLE THE UPSTREAM THOUGHTS AND ACTIONS?** If your current unhealthy behaviour is a ripple initiated by past thoughts and actions, and those thoughts or actions were traumatic or intense, you might need support figuring out the past before you can independently and productively handle the now. We all sometimes need a little extra help — we are human. Maybe you need to invest in a therapist, to call a friend or loved one, or consult your trusted religious leader. Knowing when to ask for help is a sign of strength not weakness. (Full disclosure, I could not have gotten to this place without my therapist.)

3. **WHAT IS MY FORCE MULTIPLIER?** A force multiplier is the habit or toxic thought pattern that, if changed, has an extreme positive ripple effect — a change that will give you the biggest bang for your buck. Don't expend 80 percent of your effort changing a mindset or habit that's only causing minimal distress. For example, if you eat most of your calories after eleven o'clock at night, spending

endless energy changing your breakfast will not give you extreme health results, whereas closing the fridge after eleven might. By not eating after eleven at night, you will sleep better, which will positively affect your hormones and your energy levels throughout the day. The more energetic your feel, the less likely you will be to crave sugar and the more likely you will be to go to the gym. Sleep also increases the satiation hormone leptin. When you don't get enough sleep, your body produces more ghrelin, the hunger hormone, which encourages you to crave sugar. Take a few minutes to brainstorm what your force multiplier could be.

4. **HOW DO I BE MYSELF, HONOUR MY "ME-NESS," AND HARNESS THE ASPECTS OF MY PERSONALITY TO USE MY "ME-NESS" FOR GOOD INSTEAD OF EVIL?** If you try to be someone you are not, you will eventually rebel against the new not-yours health habit. The trick is to find a way to be healthy while still embracing who you are. If you enjoy being social, great. Instead of only being social at a bar, be social while you exercise. If you hate being social, listen to music while you run, not while you sit and eat potato chips.

5. **WHAT COPING MECHANISMS AND STRATEGIES WILL BUILD MY INNER STABILITY, SELF-EFFICACY, AND SELF-WORTH?** Once you embrace your you-ness, you can find the coping mechanisms that fit your personality and work on fostering them. It is no use trying to use a strategy that will not work for you. For example, what mindset and motivational strategies will help you work out because you love yourself not because you hate yourself? For me that means telling myself I will feel better and have more energy if I train rather than focusing on how a workout will make me look.

6. **WHAT HABITS, MINDSETS, AND MOTI- VATIONAL STRATEGIES DO I HAVE THAT ARE WORTH KEEPING?** We all have unconscious inner thought loops and ingrained philosophies that lead to external health habits. The key is to become conscious of your loops, philosophies, and habits so that you can decide which loops and habits are positive and which are negative. Then work on ditching the negative and keeping the positive. Think of gathering health information as analogous to catching a baseball. Just because you catch the ball — the informa- tion — doesn't mean you have to keep or use the information. Once you have the ball you can decide what to do with it. You can decide to ditch it altogether (throw it back), hold on to it and contemplate the next move, or keep it.

7. **DO I HAVE HABITS THAT SERVE A FUNCTION, EVEN THOUGH THE OUT- COME IS UNHEALTHY?** Sometimes an unhealthy habit is married to a healthy need. Think drinking with friends, relaxing by watching TV while snacking, or eating too much at dinner as an opportunity to spend time with a spouse. Being social, relaxing, and spending time with family are all key elements of life. I would never want you to try to give those activities up to be healthy. The key is to parse the healthy need — the desire for connection with friends and family or the need for relaxation — from the less-than-ideal health choice. Can you find a way to keep the function with a healthier method? For example, if you eat too much at dinner as an opportunity to spend time with your spouse, can you instead create a habit of going for a walk together after dinner? Can you watch a movie and knit instead of eating? Go to a fun fitness class or have a cultural adventure (the art gallery, and so on) as an opportunity to catch up with friends?

MOTIVATION AND MENTAL HEALTH

Too often we frame motivation — or the lack thereof — as a discipline problem, but as I am sure most of you are well aware, it is extremely hard to motivate yourself to exercise when you feel blue. Often a lack of motivation is not a discipline problem but a mood problem.

One way out of a low mood is to move. Exercise helps to reduce anxiety, depression, tension, fatigue, and anger, and it enhances self-esteem and social bonds. The irony is that the lower your mood, the harder it is to find motivation to move. Inactivity precipitates a negative downward cycle — not moving breeds frustration, which makes you more demoralized and less motivated. The less you move the less fit you become, which makes doing everything harder, thus lowering your motivation further. The cycle continues — until you stop it.

To stop the cycle, I suggest framing exercise as a mood-management tool with everything else (weight maintenance, and so on) as a bonus. Too often we frame exercise

The worse your mood, the more important the workout. Don't wait to feel motivated to move. Move to create motivation. Move — even for just ten minutes — and you will feel better. It is the days you feel good that it is okay to skip a workout — your mood doesn't need the boost. On days you feel low, prioritize motion.

as primarily a weight-management tool — a tool to build a particular aesthetic — with the psychological effects being a bonus.

Why this reframe? There are a few reasons.

Having purely aesthetic goals may motivate you at first, but the more diverse your goals the more likely you are to stick with your program long term. Aesthetic goals often require a larger commitment of time and investment in equipment or a gym membership. The time and financial investment, not to mention the venue, can be intimidating. As soon as you frame motion as a mood-boosting tool, you legitimize the notion of small bouts of activity adding up. Even ten minutes of motion will improve your mood — and anyone can find ten minutes to exercise, especially if those ten minutes don't have to be at the gym. You can walk at work or dance around your living room.

Stating improved mood as a goal can be an excellent way in — a way to find the ignition energy to start moving. Begin referring to both starting each individual session and starting your overall health process. Once you start your ten minutes I can almost guarantee you will continue and do a few extra minutes (although even if you don't, at least you have done ten minutes). Once you start trending positive in your health, all of your little wins will domino into other wins.

The higher your overall mood the better you will be able to navigate parenthood, friendships, work life, and so on, *and* the more likely you will be to move more. Improving your mood is an excellent way to create a positive ripple effect in your overall health and well-being!

Note — and this is key — that you don't have to have a mental health disorder to actively use exercise as part of your recipe for overall psychological well-being.

Psychological well-being is analogous to physical health. Just as you shouldn't wait for a diagnosis of cardiovascular disease or diabetes to prioritize motion, you shouldn't wait to be diagnosed with a mental health disorder such as depression to work on your general mental health. Mental health also exists on a continuum; you don't need a clinical diagnosis to have an attitude of growth toward your psychological well-being.

Basically, when you feel low — when you need an extra pep in your step — move your body.

I am well aware that when you are feeling low, the "just do it" mentality is easier said than done, but believe me, it does become easier to just move once you embrace that motion can come in small chunks and can be done anywhere.

PLUG AND PLAY LIST

I suggest creating what I call a plug and play list: a list of workouts that last from two minutes to an hour. Whenever you feel blue, look at the list and figure out what you can do in the time that you have. The brilliance of the list is that you don't have to think about what to do — thinking about it wastes valuable time and cognitive energy. Instead, you just cross-reference the list to what your schedule allows and go.

One of my mom's frequent parenting lines as I grew up was "Kathleen, there is always a solution. Now let's find it." In many ways that line underpins my entire fitness philosophy. The plug and play list might just be your mood-boosting fitness solution! Here are a few suggestions to get your list started.

WHEN YOU HAVE TWO TO FIVE MINUTES:

- Dance around your living room.
- Skip.
- Do light stretching (especially if you have been sitting at your desk).
- Work your core. Try a few planks, side planks, or even a V sit in your chair at work. To do a V sit, sit tall at the front of your chair. Then lean back ten degrees. Engage your core and hold for ten-plus seconds.
- Walk up and down your stairs. Walk around the room.
- Meditate — sometimes that is even more useful than exercise.

WHEN YOU HAVE TEN MINUTES:

- Try a ten-minute workout from a fitness app.
- For ten minutes, alternate one minute of skipping (or another cardio exercise) with one minute of a multi-joint body-weight exercise (squats, lunges, and so on).
- Have a full-on dance party.
- Go for a walk around the office — say hello to your colleagues!
- Google some fun old-school aerobics moves on YouTube.

WHEN YOU HAVE FIFTEEN TO TWENTY MINUTES:

- Go for a walk — preferably outside since you have slightly more time.

- Try a yoga or body-weight routine from a fitness app.
- Try a fifteen- to twenty-minute Tabata workout. Warm up for five minutes by running on the spot or dancing around your living room. Then pick a cardio exercise (such as burpees or jumping jacks.) Do the exercise hard for twenty seconds. Rest for ten seconds. Repeat for four minutes. That is one Tabata. Try one to two more exercises. Stretch.
- Alternate one minute of skipping (or another cardio exercise) with one minute of body-weight exercises such as squats or lunges. Continue for fourteen to twenty minutes.
- Try minutes. Warm up for five minutes. Then complete one minute of a lower-body exercise, one minute of an upper-body exercise, one minute of core, and two minutes of cardio. Repeat two to three times. (See more on minutes in chapter 7.)
- Try AMRAP (as many rounds as possible). Warm up for three minutes. Then pick three strength exercises (push-ups, squats, lunges) and repeat fifteen reps of

each for eight minutes. Have some water. Pick another three exercises for your second eight-minute set. If you're doing twenty minutes, repeat a third set of four minutes. Stretch.

WHEN YOU HAVE THIRTY MINUTES OR MORE:

- Try a longer AMRAP. Warm up for five minutes. Then pick three body-weight exercises and repeat fifteen reps of each for ten minutes. Have some water. Pick another three exercises for your second ten-minute set. Stretch.
- Go for a run or walk and include a few intervals. For example, try mini pick-ups. After a warm-up, alternate fifteen seconds fast with forty-five seconds regular.
- Try a longer minutes workout. Warm up for five minutes. Then complete one minute of a lower-body exercise, one minute of an upper-body exercise, one minute of core, and two minutes of cardio. Repeat four times. Stretch.
- Once you have forty-five minutes you can really fit in a full strength workout. Try circuit-style weights,

a workout class (on an app, at the gym, or on YouTube), or alternating five minutes of all-out cardio with ten minutes of multi-joint strength exercises.

When possible, don't simply match the workout to your time frame; also match the workout to your mood. If you're feeling angry, you might attend a boxing class — get out your aggression. If you're feeling tense, consider downloading a short at-home meditation or yoga workout. Feeling low? I suggest some cardio — dance, skip, or go for a run.

The key is that you can choose how to use your body, and since exercise positively effects mood, you can choose to change your mood. As with all things to do with your health, know your triggers and always have a strategy (a plan A) but know you can recalibrate and try your plan B if needed. For example, I know live media makes me slightly nervous, so I try to always schedule a good workout before a TV segment to kill my butterflies. If I can't do a full workout I do some burpees and jumping jacks before I shower and change for the show. I know me. I know what I need. Figure out what you need and do that. Tweak the Scout motto slightly: Always be prepared but be prepared knowing both who you are now and who you want your future self to be.

MINDSET TAKE-OFF

· ·

You are ready for mindset take-off. You now know how critical a positive internal dialogue is. You know awareness brings choice. You know to be yourself. You have answered the seven key mindset questions. (If you haven't, go back and answer those.) You know you can change your mood through motion. You are now ready to create your MINDSETmix.

STAYING MOTIVATED IN THE PROCESS

Establishing a positive inner dialogue means letting go of unproductive, toxic thoughts — letting go of the goal of perfection. In doing so, you detach much of the meaning connected to actions and choices. The result? Non-judgmental reactions — productively rerouting your GPS.

This process can feel exhausting. I get that. To stay motivated, consider embracing the goal of feeding the wolf you want to win. There is an ancient story of a grandmother sitting with her granddaughter describing two wolves in battle. One wolf is angry and filled with resentment and unproductive thoughts. The other wolf is thoughtful, filled with love and compassion for himself and others; his thoughts are productive and habits healthy. When the grandchild asks which wolf will win the fight, the grandmother answers, "The one you feed."

Think of your thought patterns like the wolves. The wolf you should feed is the thought pattern you want your future self to hold. If you want the future you to make healthier, more productive decisions, feed that wolf; make yourself think and act differently so that your healthier, happier wolf flourishes.

Let go of punitive or belittling tones. Learn how to talk to yourself in the language that will best serve you. Work to

I am constantly fascinated that my current self has self-compassion, yet hardly ever falls off the health horse. The younger Kathleen assumed one needed tough love to stay accountable; the alternative to beating oneself up would be coddling and pandering to desires. The older Kathleen knows there are many options between pandering and self-hate or shame. Having compassion does not mean forgoing growth and positive actions. Far from it. In my twenties I was unproductively hard on myself. My current self has few toxic thoughts. The result? Fewer unhealthy habits; I speak respectfully to myself and, behold, I make better decisions.

form an internal dialogue that you would be proud for your child, best friend, spouse, or parent to have. Love yourself. Period.

Think globally about your health — not myopically; all your actions and thoughts work together. Don't make one healthy choice so you can justify other unhealthy choices. Own all your choices. Embrace that the longer you have held a habit, the longer it will take to replace. Lean in to non-judgmental observation of yourself and your actions. Instead of metaphorically flogging yourself, work to create a strong sense of self; the stronger your inner dialogue, the easier it will be to adapt appropriately and reroute when life gets in the way.

As you read through the strategies in chapter 9, remember that the trick is to not only parse what you think might work for you, but not to get caught up in "analysis paralysis." Instead of constantly getting caught up in grand — sometimes ineffable — futures, focus on what positive step you can make in this moment. Really, the only moment we have control over is now. If we want to control the future, we have to control the now. Instead of feeling overwhelmed by an all-or-nothing understanding of fitness, ask yourself what small thing you could do now. Could you go for a walk? Drink a glass of water? Crack a smile? Even brainstorming how you might get off the sofa next time is a step in the right direction. In MINDSETmix creation embracing the now means just try something. If it doesn't work, try something else. The key — as I have said many times and will continue to hammer home — is to start. If you don't start, you have nothing to tweak.

Embrace the Now

• • • • • • • • • • •

Life is simply a series of "now moments." When possible, make the "now" something you enjoy. When enjoyment is too much to ask, make the moment one filled with integrity; act in a way your future self would be proud of. When integrity evades you, be present in the moment so you can at least note the interaction and thus learn how to respond rather than react to the situation.

Strategies for Your MINDSETmix

*A useful **MINDSETmix** requires the creation of a strong individualized internal dialogue. We all have moments of low motivation. What keeps me from eating badly and bailing on a workout? Self-talk! Especially useful, snappy internal hashtags.*

Welcome to chapter 9 — the second of the MINDSETmix chapters. In this chapter I will take you through a variety of mindset strategies — it is your job to figure out the combination of elements from various strategies that will work for you. Think of the strategies as an à la carte menu; instead of picking one dish, pick elements of all the different dishes to create your meal. If you get stumped while creating your mix, refer back to the seven questions you answered in chapter 8. The answers will offer valuable insight and inform the creation of your MINDSETmix.

Regardless of the MINDSETmix you create, another key skill to develop is the skill of talking to yourself; all MINDSETmixes require the creation of a productive, purposeful, individualized internal dialogue.

We all have moments of low motivation. You may love exercise but still sometimes want to bail on a workout. How can you stop yourself from making poor choices?

Self-talk tailored to addressing your individual triggers, pitfalls, negative internal dialogue, negative brain propaganda, and goals. Prepare yourself to deal with the inevitable low-motivation moments. (There is that word again — *preparation*.)

You have to tailor your internal dialogue to your low moments — when your co-worker brings in homemade treats or you're exhausted after work and just want pizza and your sofa. It is not enough to figure out an individualized program for the motivated you — you don't really need self-talk when you're already motivated. You need self-talk when you are tired, have a low mood, are angry, or are overwhelmed — when you are your most vulnerable self.

Remember the pause — the purposeful moment you take between being stimulated and your response? Figure out what will be best said in moments when you need the pause — when you want extra helpings you don't need, when you want to skip a workout, or when you want to ditch your healthier plan in favour of a more fun plan.

When I don't want to train, I say, "Kathleen, you always feel better when you move. Moving is not a punishment; it is a privilege. If you don't want to do your entire workout, fine, but you have to do something. Something is always better than nothing. Just start."

Consider distilling your self-talk into nuggets or mottos — or what I jokingly refer to as internal hashtags — that are easy to remember and repeat. Here are a few of my favourites:

➡ #IAmWorthyOfSelfCare
➡ #TheWorseYourMoodThe More ImportantTheWorkout
➡ #PerfectionIsTheOpposite OfDONE
➡ #blahblahblahGoWORKOUT

Identify the roadblocks keeping you from succeeding. Then strategize your targeted self-talk for that situation. Form the internal dialogue that will be of best use to you. Remember, only after mindset changes can behavioural changes occur.

MINDSETMIX STRATEGY 1: PRIORITIZE SLEEP

Sleep fosters resilience, strengthens your say no muscle, and increases motivation.

It is almost impossible to make healthy decisions and to motivate yourself to stay away from sugar, reduce caffeine, or go to the gym when you are exhausted. A sleep deficit causes a ripple effect that potentially affects *all* health decisions. When I give in to sugar, I am nine times out of ten exhausted — my resilience is low and my say no muscle non-existent. When rested, healthy choices don't feel as forced.

Adequate sleep should be a non-negotiable. Sleeping will increase alertness,

mental clarity, and energy, not to mention regulate your weight. Sleeping helps your body and brain recover and regulates the hormones that control your appetite. When you don't get enough sleep, your body produces more ghrelin, the hunger hormone. Ghrelin encourages you to crave sweets. In contrast, getting enough sleep encourages your body to produce more leptin. Leptin will help you feel full. Too many of us are far too willing to give up a few hours of sleep in favour of watching TV, working, or socializing. Making one healthy choice, like working out, is not a justification to sacrifice sleep; healthy choices should

---

Healthy Sleep Routines

Wanting to sleep and actually being able to sleep are often two different things. Consider implementing a pre-bedtime relaxation routine.

Turn off all screens at least thirty minutes before bed. In that thirty minutes try having a bath — an Epsom salt bath can be especially relaxing — or meditating. Do some deep breathing, gentle yoga, or stretching, or lie lengthwise on a foam roller.

complement each other, not become justifications for alternative actions. No one — not even the most A-type competitive athletic gym bunny — can thrive without sleep. A lack of sleep is — sometimes literally — a form of torture.

MINDSETMIX STRATEGY 2: FIGURE OUT YOUR UNIQUE FLAVOUR OF SELF-SABOTAGE

Self-sabotage is the mindset and negative brain propaganda that we use to justify unhealthy choices. We all have our own flavour of self-sabotage. The trick is to identify your unique flavour and figure out ways to best manage it.

Self-Sabotage Flavour I: Rationalizing with the Snowball Effect

Missing one workout is not the same as missing five workouts. One cookie is not the same as seven. One glass of wine is not the same as the bottle. Too many of us let ourselves snowball; we rationalize missing a workout or eating multiple treats by telling ourselves that the damage has already been done, so why not indulge further?

Why not? Portions count and all movement adds up. Mindfully eating small portions of indulgences we love is a healthy part of life. Mindless binges are not physically or psychologically healthy. You can easily recover from missing one workout or eating a piece of dark chocolate. A week of workouts and twenty pieces of chocolate are another story.

We are only human. Setting the unrealistic expectation that you will never have another treat or miss a workout simply sets one up for failure. The trick is, to quote Arianna Huffington in her interview on *The Tim Ferriss Show* in October 2017, to "course correct" as quickly as possible. When you feel you are self-sabotaging say to yourself, "Course correct." Or, "You're swivelling." Your future self will be happier if you don't have another cookie. The lesson is that small indulgences are a healthy part of life; you can compensate for them by going for a walk or eating more vegetables the following day. If you let that one choice snowball into multiple indulgences it will take days (even weeks) to get back on track.

We all sometimes let choices snowball. I know I have. The thing is, when you take the time to analyze the practice, you realize how absurd and counterproductive it is. Imagine spilling a small amount of mustard on your shirt and then saying, "Since I spilt this much, I might as well spill the entire bottle on myself … or better yet,

pour a bath of mustard and roll around in it." That is not helpful and neither is letting yourself have multiple cookies just because you had one.

Self-Sabotage Flavour 2: Trying to Fit a Square Peg in a Round Hole

Adopting a method of change that doesn't fit your personality is a surefire way to fail. Other people's health and diet regimens

---

The Top Two Tiers of the Cake

• • • • • • • • • • •

When I am tempted to let one unhealthy choice snowball into five or six, I remember an image of a tiered cake I found in a book by Judith Beck. Imagine a wedding cake with food choices written on each tier. Each tier represents an amount of food consumed in a sitting.

The top and smallest tier has something like a one hundred–calorie cookie written in it. In each lower tier the choices get more extravagant. The next tier might include two cookies, a piece of cake, and a hot chocolate that, if eaten, would total 800 calories. By the final tier — the bottom layer — there are thousands of calories of food listed within the box.

If you let one choice snowball, it will take time to get back on track. Aim to only ever eat the top tier of the cake and take the time to actually enjoy the food you are consuming.

are exactly that — theirs. Sure, you can twist yourself into knots and adapt to someone else's program for a few weeks, but chances are you won't be able to maintain the program over the long haul. Adopt a method of change and a lifestyle regimen realistic for you.

For example, if you know you are most successful when you implement changes gradually — the small changes add up camp — try my weekly add-on method described in chapter 2. If you like radical change — if big changes make you feel in control — try the 180 daily pyramid method for change from chapter 2.

Self-Sabotage Flavour 3: Crying Wolf

Crying wolf refers to constantly reverting to the had-to excuse. "Had-to" puts the locus of control external to yourself. Sure, once in a small while unhealthy choices are unavoidable — life is unpredictable — but most of the time, if we set ourselves up for success, we can plan so that healthy habits are possible. Had-to statements should be the exception, not the norm. When you constantly have to make bad choices you can't ever legitimately let

yourself off the hook when life really gets in the way — you can't trust your internal barometer.

Do these sentences sound familiar?

- "I had to skip a workout because of X."
- "I had to eat fast food because it was all that was available."
- "I had to have frozen pizza because I had no other food in the house."

If had-to is your go-to, then crying wolf is your method of self-sabotage.

Crying wolf is counterproductive. It does not allow for a growth mindset or consistent healthy choices and, even worse, lying to yourself does not foster self-trust, hope, or self-respect.

Accountability is key. You will never achieve your goals if you don't hold yourself accountable. An alternative to had-to — which assumes an external locus of control — might be something like, I did not plan in advance, and thus this less-than-ideal choice has become what is available. When you own an unhealthy choice, you at least potentially learn from the experience — growth is always valuable. Adopting a passive voice — the had-to voice — is unproductive; you can't learn from a had-to stance.

Had-to crying wolf statements do not build self-trust (see chapter 10 for more on self-trust). How can you trust yourself if you are constantly misrepresenting the truth to yourself and others? Own your choices. Most of the time some variation of a healthy choice is possible. The freeing result of honesty is, when you are honest with yourself — and thus have self-trust — then the few times you do actually legitimately have to make a less-than-ideal choice you can easily forget about it. The irony is, by owning all your choices — the good and the bad — you can be more self-compassionate about what you actually don't have control over.

To lose weight, help lower blood pressure, improve energy, or decrease anxiety, you need to change your preferences and daily habits so that more often than not you make healthy choices. Working out once per month and abstaining from cake once per week, although possibly a step in the right direction, will not result in you reaching your long-term goals. Consistency is key.

Trust in self (integrity) and consistency are both paramount when working to achieve a healthier lifestyle.

How can you avoid crying wolf? Stop saying you had to! Set yourself up for health success.

- **MAKE YOUR HEALTHY HABITS CONVENIENT AND YOUR UNHEALTHY HABITS UTTERLY INCONVENIENT.** Orchestrate your life so that it is easy to make healthy choices and harder to make unhealthy ones (so you don't have to reach for the chocolate bar). Feeling hungry, exhausted, angry, sad, or thirsty lowers resilience, which means it takes more energy and resolve to make a healthy choice. Instead of being surprised by your physiological needs and emotions — we all get tired and hungry — normalize this aspect of life and take the necessary preemptive steps, such as carrying healthy snacks.

- **ENSURE YOUR WORKOUT LENGTH, LOCATION, AND TIMING ARE REALISTIC FOR YOUR SCHEDULE.** For example, I completed a Muay Thai Sweat Test review in July 2017 for the *Globe and Mail*. I liked the workout but, at almost two hours, it is not realistic for my schedule. I know, for me, if I ever decide to do martial arts, I will do a martial arts fitness-based workout (they tend to be shorter) or work with a trainer one-on-one. Yes, the Muay Thai class was awesome, but I won't benefit if I know I will never make myself go.

- **USE FUTURE "IF … THEN" STATEMENTS.** Decide in advance — when you are level-headed — what you will do when your future self wants to deviate from your health plan. Create "if … then" statements regarding how you will handle any health landmines. For example, if I want to eat a treat at a party, then I will make myself wait 15 minutes. If I decide to indulge after 15 minutes, then I will restrict myself to a thumb-sized portion. Or, if I want to eat in front of the TV, then I will knit instead.

- **CHANGE YOUR LANGUAGE.** Don't use language that undermines self-efficacy. Frame experiences with a can-do attitude; use words that give you the most amount of self-control, hope, and positive forward momentum. *Can't* externalizes your locus of control — and potentially sends you into a downward shame spiral. At least with

"I decided not to," you own your choices. Ask yourself, When will I work out? not Will I work out? Say, "I get to exercise" not "I have to exercise." Or, if you are not motivated by the idea of exercising, but like the idea of dancing, frame your workout as taking a dance class.

- **BE SPECIFIC.** Generalized excuses lead to generalized solutions. Replace "I am under stress" with "I am feeling stressed by my family in X ways." My mother always said, "Find solutions not excuses." The trouble is, until you determine the problem, you can't figure out a solution. Pinpoint specific problems. Figure out targeted solutions.

- **STOP TELLING YOURSELF YOU ARE TOO BUSY.** "I don't have time" is the grown-up equivalent of "the dog ate my homework." Do you use the too busy excuse because you are trying to commit to a plan you hate? Are you too busy because you are afraid of failure and therefore don't want to try? Are you too busy because you haven't taken the time to rearrange your schedule? The key is preparation, preparation, preparation. Of course you are too busy to work out if you haven't carved out the time. Schedule in your workouts and analyze your upcoming week so you can troubleshoot possible problems and come up with solutions.

- **MAKE MOVEMENT FUN**. If you hate something, you will always find other more important ways to use your time! Instead, make exercise palatable. Make a date with a friend or sign up for adult dance classes.

- **YOU ARE AN ADULT — OWN YOUR CHOICES**. If you decide not to exercise, fine. But say something like, "I decided not to exercise today because I made something else a priority." Deciding not to exercise is okay sometimes — but acknowledge that it was a choice and understand that there is a cost. When you are legitimately too busy to spend two hours getting to and from the gym, figure out how you can weave motion into your day. Everyone has time to take the stairs instead of the escalator. Do squats

and lunges as you watch your children practise their sport, walk your kids to school then jog or run home, or pace as you take conference calls. Everyone can pepper movement throughout their day.

- **REPLACE "I AM TOO BUSY" WITH "MOVEMENT IS A NON-NEGOTIABLE!"** Exercise is not an if; it's a when. If you let it, life will always take over, so don't let it! Commit to figuring out how to integrate some motion into every day of your life. There is no perfect week to start training; just put on your running shoes and go out for a walk!

Self-Sabotage Flavour 4: The World Is Not Fair

Stop focusing on the negatives. Too many of us self-sabotage by constantly focusing on what we can't change and what we don't have. We are the perpetual Negative Adolescent Nelly: Imagine a child in the schoolyard who, when she doesn't get her way, instead of working out the problem — sharing, communicating, being mature, and so on — simply takes her ball and goes home. These thought patterns are not productive. The child desperately wants a play friend but would rather be hurt and alone than vulnerable and communicative. The child simply hangs on to the negative — the can'ts — rather than working to find a solution.

Too many adults do this with food and exercise. They desperately want to be healthier, but when they encounter something that is not fair or hit an emotional or a physical roadblock, instead of responding and finding solutions, they react and focus on the negatives; they react to their vulnerability with a Negative Nelly attitude of can't and won't and I deserve that treat. They take their ball and they go home. The problem is, just as this action doesn't get the child the end result they wanted — a new friend — it also does not result in the adult making healthier choices. Negative, reactive, unfair self-talk is unproductive.

Seth Godin, in his interview on *The Tim Ferriss Show* podcast in February 2016, refers to this type of mindset as the "sour mindset" — we are not getting what we "deserve" (we deserve cake and easy weight loss) or the world is not fair (why weren't we born skinny?). Stop with "I deserve" — that simply leads to unhealthy choices such as "I went for a thirty-minute run today so I deserve the beer, cake, fried food, or [fill in the blank]." You are not five negotiating with your mom to stay up past your bedtime. You are an adult. What you "deserve" is to love yourself enough to make healthy choices. Stop with the "world hates me" negative attitude — even if it were true (spoiler alert: it's not), it is not helpful; it is self-limiting.

Your body is not a garbage can — put healthy food into it. Portion sizes are always important, even on days you exercise. Functionality, strength, energy, and athletic ability are important. Work out to feel strong and empowered. Use your body or lose your body. Even if you work out, prolonged sitting negatively affects the cardiovascular, lymphatic, and digestive systems, not to mention your metabolism. Your health — in its totality — is key. Instead of creating an inventory of what you can't have and what you can't do, inventory your successes. Learn from any missteps. Course correct quickly.

Who says the world should always be fair and nice to you? Being healthy is not always roses and fairy tales — but healthy choices are still healthy choices and negative, unproductive "I deserve" self-talk is not helpful. Period.

Focus on what you do have and what you can do. I am not arguing for blind positivity — this is not about being glass half empty or glass half full — this is about embracing that life takes work, that life is not fair, and most critically that the only moment we have control over is the now. Stop sabotaging your efforts by automatically always going negative — by focusing on what you don't have and you can't do. Focus on what you can do in that moment that will be a positive step in the right direction. If you like the glass metaphor, instead of focusing on what is already in the glass, think, What can I do to fill my glass?

MINDSETMIX STRATEGY 3: FIND YOUR HACKS

Motivation is made, not found. If you're having trouble making yourself move, rethink your motivational strategies. Adopt a fitness hack. *Hacks* are innovative ways to motivate or trick yourself into getting over your hang-ups and making healthy choices.

Harness the aspect of each hack that allows you to use your own nature for good instead of evil. If you're competitive, instead of betting on sports, join a sports team. If you enjoy organizing everyone else's life, put together a workout group. If you like cooking, research healthy recipes. If you're frugal, find ways to save money by cooking healthy food at home. If you love TV, replace sitting on the sofa with TV time on the treadmill.

Always have a growth mindset; recognize what has and has not worked for you. Capitalize on what has worked. If buying fitness clothes motivates you, do that. Learn from what has not worked. If you aim to work out in the morning but consistently snooze the alarm, figure out why you are tired (do you need to go to bed earlier?) or decide to work out at an alternative time.

Kathleen-Approved Fitness Hacks

- **COUPLE EXERCISE WITH SOMETHING YOU ENJOY.** Watch TV or listen to a podcast, an audiobook, or music as you work out. Better yet, have a program you are only allowed to listen to or watch when exercising.

- **GET A FITNESS BUDDY.** Friends make everything more fun. You are less likely to skip a workout if you are meeting someone. Meet your buddy and do fun fitness classes, go for a walk, do fun partner strength exercises at the gym, or simply meet and do cardio on side-by-side machines. With my friends, I do everything from yoga to barre to boxing. Then we go get a tea and catch up.

- **REWARD YOURSELF.** Set goals and non-food-related rewards: a hot bubble bath, a new workout outfit, or a movie with friends. Don't let yourself have the reward if you don't reach your goal.

- **FIND SOMEONE WHO INSPIRES YOU AND LEARN FROM THEM.** This could be someone from your real life or someone on social media. No one who is successful succeeds the first time. Try sending a message to your social media guru, or ask the person who inspires you in real life how they overcame obstacles. Then extrapolate and apply their experiences to your own life.

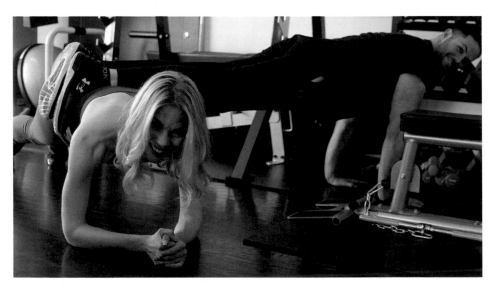

Plank fun with my friend and colleague Harry Scott.

- **CREATE UNIQUE STRATEGIES FOR SUCCESS**. Working out in the morning? Sleep in your exercise clothes. Have an unpredictable schedule? Always have a gym bag packed and ready to go. One of my clients gets up and puts her sports bra overtop of her night clothes and then hops on her treadmill. She knows that if she stops to change she will skip her workout.

- **CREATE FRIENDLY COMPETITION.** Figure out what drives you. If you care about saving money, pay yourself every time you train. When you reach a pre-established amount, splurge on something you normally wouldn't buy. If competing with others is more your jam, sign up for ClassPass or a virtual activity tracker; compete with friends on how many classes you attend or how many steps you take.

- **CREATE VISUAL REMINDERS OF YOUR SUCCESS.** Have a calendar on the fridge and place a sticker on it every time you exercise, or create a spreadsheet or graph and record your workouts.

- **MAKE EXERCISE *FUN* IN ANY WAY POSSIBLE.** Join a fancy gym so you feel special. Don't like fancy? Join a sports team or a running group so that working out becomes a social experience. Figure out what drives you, then do that.

It's Not the Final Coin

· · · · · · · · · ·

When it comes to your health, remember that all of your small choices add up. Think of it as analogous to the parable of the final coin that makes one wealthy. The prior coins are what makes the final coin significant. The coins are analogous to steps in your health journey. To get anywhere important takes many steps. That final step only puts you over the finish line if you have taken the preceding steps. Keep going!

MINDSETMIX STRATEGY 4: FOSTER MINDFULNESS

By *foster mindfulness*, I mean foster purposeful awareness. We all make innumerable daily health choices, most of which are based on internal thought loops, inner dialogues, habits, and actions we are not even aware of. Actions are unquestioned, unconscious — part of the fabric of our existence. The only way to make a future change is to become aware of the now. There are many ways to foster mindfulness. Here are some strategies you might find useful.

Journal

Journaling can help highlight the disconnect between the health choices we think we make and the choices we actually make, as well as the reasons behind our choices.

Record food choices, portions, alcohol and water consumption, as well as emotions and intentions behind your food choices. You can stress eat or binge out of loneliness on any diet — lots of people overeat gluten-free cake and paleo treats. If you don't become aware of the what, why, and how of your eating patterns, your personal food habits follow you from nutrition program to nutrition program.

A favourite twist on the classic food journal is the X versus O variation. This iteration can be a helpful way to gain an understanding of your emotions in relation to food. Draw five circles on each page of a journal. Each page represents one day, and the five circles represent three meals and two snacks. After every meal ask yourself, Did I stop eating when I was full and did I generally make healthy choices? If the answer is yes, you don't have to write down what you ate; simply put an X through the circle. If you made food choices that you were not happy with, write down what you ate, as well as how and why you ate the food. Were you tired or depressed? Did you grab food mindlessly off your co-worker's desk or eat as you cooked? Hopefully your week will be full of Xs, but if it's not, figure out when and why you made your unhealthy choices. Decide how you can make better choices next time.

Become a Purist

It is almost impossible to be mindful of portions and food choices when you mix activities. How can you pay attention to your choices while standing, scarfing food off a colleague's desk, watching TV, eating to ward off boredom in a meeting, or nibbling while cooking? So become a purist and focus on one thing at a time.

- **EAT WHEN YOU EAT.** And do only that. Stop eating when you are driving, standing, watching TV, cooking, or working at a computer. Multi-tasking might have its positives, but eating should never be a multi-tasked activity. Savour your food. Appreciate the flavours. Give your brain the opportunity to tell you, "Stop, I am full."

- **DON'T STAND AND EAT.** Don't mindlessly eat while you are cooking, during meetings, or while socializing at a party. Make snacking while cooking off limits — non-negotiable. Often, by the time the cook sits down to dinner they have already consumed at least half a meal's worth of food.

- **AT PARTIES, DRINK WATER** throughout the night so that your hands stay occupied and you don't become dehydrated. Before you put anything in your mouth ask yourself if you really want it. Before I nibble on party snacks, I try to remember to ask myself, "Kathleen, will your future self be happy that you consumed this?" If the answer is no, I try not to pick up the food.

- **STOP EATING IN FRONT OF THE TV.** Instead of nibbling while you watch TV, drink water or do an activity that keeps your hands busy, like knitting. When I want to snack in front of the TV, I try to distract myself by using the foam roller or stretching.

- **PUT YOUR FORK DOWN BETWEEN BITES.** Don't hoover down your food. Slow down; savour the flavours. Enjoy your meal and the company you are with.

MINDSETMIX STRATEGY 5:
MAKE CHOICES AS IF FOR A LOVED ONE

After almost twenty years in the health field, I have noticed a distinct pattern. Too often there is a disconnect between what clients think is good enough for their loved ones and what is good enough for them personally. Too many people (especially mothers) are able to outline in detail the healthy choices they make for others, but find it nearly impossible to implement the same choices for themselves.

I now suggest that clients with this tendency consciously choose to make decisions as if they were making them for someone else. The strategy works because it makes you mindful — you can't just swipe food off your co-worker's desk; you have to stop and think about the consequences of your health decisions.

 For the next month I dare you to make all your health choices as if you were making them for someone you care deeply for — an elderly parent, your child, or in my case a client. Schedule your workouts as if you were scheduling a child's activities. Pack snacks as if you were packing snacks for your child or an elderly parent. Give yourself a bedtime and strong morning routines — as you would a child. Talk constructively to yourself — with compassion and a goal of growth and learning — as if you were parenting a child; look for barriers and solutions, critique the individual problem rather than denigrating you as a person. Speak in a friendly tone. See what happens.

- **SCHEDULE YOUR LIFE LIKE YOU WOULD A CHILD'S LIFE.** Most parents I meet actively plan their children's activity schedule; they know that if they don't schedule in movement, their kids will sit and play video games or do something equally inactive. Unfortunately, they often don't actively schedule and prioritize their own exercise regimen. The key word is *actively* — schedule your activity like you would your child's. If it is not in the schedule it won't happen.

- **APPLY THE SAME AMOUNT OF MIND-FULNESS** to your own nutrition as you would for a loved one. You wouldn't expect your kids (or someone you care about) to eat food off of your plate, snack before dinner, or mindlessly grab a chocolate bar at three in the afternoon, but that is how many parents I work with feed themselves.

- **TALK TO YOURSELF IN A WAY YOU WOULD WANT** your child or best friend to talk about themselves. Too often clients confess to an

Become aware of more than just your nutrition choices; become mindful of your exercise and sleep habits, your internal self-talk, and even the people you surround yourself with.

Love yourself enough to make healthy, nutritionally dense food choices with the same diligence you would for a child or an elderly parent.

unhealthy internal dialogue — that they are fat and unlovable, and so on — and then in the same hour discuss how worried they are about their children's negative body image. Get rid of your destructive internal dialogue. You wouldn't let your best friend or child talk badly about their body and self-worth; why is it okay for you to berate yourself?

If you're not a parent and don't have an elderly dependent, and thus the idea of living how you would want your child or parent to live is not helpful, find another way to apply this concept. We all have people we care about; aim to apply the same standards to self-care as you apply when caring for your loved ones.

MINDSETMIX STRATEGY 6: TRY HABIT SUBSTITUTION VERSUS HABIT CHANGING

Overhauling multiple eating and lifestyle habits at once can feel overwhelming and complicated. For many — especially the small changes add up camp — it is easier to keep a current habit but substitute the content of the habit. Substituting healthier options, but keeping the habit, is a way to give your taste buds and life rhythms time to adjust.

Instead of changing the habit — the action — substitute the content.

Instead of replacing your dog walk with a gym workout, make the walk a workout. Instead of replacing TV time, exercise while you watch TV. Or instead of trying to not have pasta, have pasta, but have bean pasta rather than white, nutritionally vapid pasta. Have cereal, just have a low-sugar variation. Enjoy your coffee, but find substitutions for the sugar. Find ways to tweak your existing life rhythms for maximum health returns.

See chapter 4 for some Kathleen-approved healthy substitutions.

OWNING YOUR MINDSETMIX

There are many strategies you could use to create your MINDSETmix, now it is your job to decide which strategy works for you. As we discussed when creating your NUTRITIONmix and WORKOUTmix, something can be theoretically excellent but still not right for you. Yes, all of these mindset strategies are excellent in theory, but the theory is moot unless it works for you. For example, I find telling myself, "You just have to start. If you need to stop after ten minutes you can," extremely helpful. Once I start I never actually take the out. That said, I know many of my triathlete friends who find that motivational strategy counterproductive — if they give themselves an out they will take it. My strategy is not better than theirs. I move. They move.

I aim for healthy striving and productive self-reflection rather than perfection. This allows me to respond appropriately rather than react emotionally. That said, my health quest is just that — mine.

Figure out what will make your future self happier, healthier, self-confident, self-trusting, and present. If you're thinking, I am still not sure what makes me happy, let alone how to build self-trust and appropriate responses, don't worry! This is common. So many of us are disconnected; we don't know who we are and thus what would give us joy or how to trust ourselves and react appropriately.

I have been there. As my therapist has said to me, you have to know what you want before you can make it happen. I have follow-through, but the younger Kathleen struggled to identify what she wanted and thus what I should follow through on. Full disclosure: I am still working on figuring out joy and self-trust — if you figure it out, please email me! — but I have come a long way over the past few years.

The MINDSETmix that works for me combines a few chosen fitness hacks — training with a fitness buddy, trying to make fitness fun, aiming to make choices as if I am making them for a loved one, and, most critically, always owning my choices. I make it a point to never cry wolf. If I make a less-than-ideal choice I own it. I decide that the choice was worth it and productive (for example, eating a moderate portion of something I love is actually healthier than absolute deprivation — life is short) or that the choice was unproductive. If I deem the choice unproductive, I aim to learn from it so I can make a better choice next time. Either way, the choice was mine.

All that matters is that, in both scenarios, we are getting the job done; we do that by finding strategies that work for us.

I have found the three mixes that work for me — at least the current me. The foundation of my NUTRITIONmix is that I am always aware of what I put in my mouth and how I am feeling. If I choose to make an unhealthy choice, fine, but it is always an active choice. My WORKOUTmix is prefaced on thinking of daily motion is a when not an if; the worse my mood and the more highly sensitized my reactions, the more I push myself to move. My MINDSETmix includes listening to self-improvement, educational, and self-help audiobooks and podcasts. Listening — then translating the information into applicable nuggets — helps me stay grounded, happy, perspective-filled, and trending positive. Last, I commit daily to having a growth mindset — always non-judgmentally analyzing my actions.

When you want to make an unhealthy choice, consider talking yourself through how you will feel depending on the choice you make. The unhealthy choice might feel good in the moment, but consider how you will feel in three hours. For example, when I want to skip a workout I tell myself, "Yes, if I skip my workout I can relax, but the quality of my relaxation time will be compromised." I will be metaphorically kicking myself. On the flip side, if I am active, even for twenty minutes, I will enjoy relaxing. Plus, I will feel great. My entire day will be better. Never forget that good things take time. Adopting a healthier lifestyle takes perseverance.

Perseverance is hard. Adopting a healthier lifestyle can feel overwhelming. Creating your three mixes — getting on your health horse — is in many ways the easy part. You stay on your health horse by knowing that we all fall off the horse — we all fail. The trick is to course correct as quickly as possible. You have to get back on your horse ASAP. That process involves self-trust, self-compassion, and the ability to respond rather than react. More on all three concepts in chapter 10.

Staying on Your Health Horse

You're almost at the end! You now have the tools to create your realistic and individualized NUTRITIONmix, WORKOUTmix, and MINDSETmix. Congratulations!

Sure, designing the mixes is one thing, but now you may be wondering how to keep it all going. It is time to work on a few key skills: self-trust (which includes self-compassion) and the ability to respond appropriately (rather than react) to health stimuli.

The unfortunate truth is that — no matter how amazing your mixes — you will fall off of your health horse at some point.

When you fall, it is imperative that you know how to get back up! You may have made an A+ mix, but your process will still involve ups and downs.

As T.S. Eliot wrote in his 1940 poem "East Coker," "There is only the trying." In Kathleen-speak "the trying" means "the process." So think, *There is only the process.* It is key to embrace the process in large part because the process is the now, and the now — as opposed to the end result — is what you have absolute control over. One of the keys to life is to focus on what you can control rather than what you can't control.

It is also important to embrace the process because once you conceptualize health as a process you can appreciate that your health journey will not be linear.

Life is never one note but involves ups and downs; it is unrealistic to expect your health to be any different — your health is not divorced from your life. Your process will include morose days, days when you feel burdened with a general sense of malaise, days when you feel on top of the world, days when you feel irritable and highly sensitive, days when you feel angry, days when you make multiple less-than-ideal health choices, and days when you kick health ass — and that is okay. To be successful in health (and life) you have to have the capacity to navigate the undulations that are inherent to every process.

I am giving you permission to fail at all of your mixes as many times as you need to — as long as you keep getting back on your horse. There are caveats: do not conflate not trying with trying and failing (you have to be on the horse to fall); and through every failure, work on fostering self-compassion, self-trust, and the ability to respond appropriately.

UNDERSTANDING APPROPRIATE RESPONSES

The skill that needs to overlay every mix — so that you can actually stay on your horse — is an ability to appropriately respond (versus react) to health stimuli. Your ability to respond appropriately is inextricably linked to self-trust and self-compassion.

Appropriate responses are productive; they are measured, value-driven, rational, solution-based, and conscious. When you respond appropriately, you don't delude yourself, but you also don't make something a bigger deal than it needs to be. You don't catastrophize. You don't self-sabotage by buying into all-or-nothing health binaries. You don't sort yourself into either bad and unhealthy or good and healthy. You see things for what they are. If you make an unhealthy choice you analyze that specific situation rather than generalizing the problem to an overall character flaw. You don't give in to negative brain propaganda. Your response toolbox includes more than the extreme ends of the health-reaction spectrum of anger, shame, and belittling self-talk or self-pandering and coddling.

Respond appropriately is another way of saying apply basic critical thinking skills to your health. In theory, this is easy. In reality, it's very challenging. If making rational health decisions came naturally, we would all sit less, move more, and eat fresh fruits and vegetables daily.

Visualize a response (not a reaction) as an individual lying comfortably in a

I have been mulling over and writing on the concept of appropriate responses, self-trust, self-love, and compassion for years. I often write about issues I personally find challenging, and until now I couldn't figure out why moderation and self-acceptance were so hard for me. While writing *Your Fittest Future Self*, I had an epiphany. I have been understanding self-love, self-trust, and appropriate and moderate responses as separate concepts. They are not.

What I now know is that the ability to respond appropriately is inextricably linked to one's level of self-trust. Put another way, I struggle with liking myself, being temperate in goal setting, and moderate in actions. Rules are easy for me. The slippery slope of moderation is a whole other — extremely scary — ballgame. Rules have been my bunker of health safety, providing me a facade of certainty in the very uncertain and scary world of making health decisions. The more I trust myself, the less scary the world is.

Making appropriate responses will feel organic — less forced — as I learn to trust myself. I won't be as petrified of moderation — of letting myself live in the grey area — once I trust that I won't slide down the side of the mountain. Or to take more of a growth-mindset approach, I will be less afraid of moderation once I know that if I do slide slightly, I can pull myself back to safety and learn from the slip.

hammock strung up between two extremes. Appropriate responses exist in that middle ground; they can only occur when one holds a rational, growth-oriented, compassion-filled mindset. Now, yes, everyone's middle ground will be unique — my health middle ground is most people's version of extreme — but, as I keep reiterating, individualization is a good thing. It does not matter what your favourite celebrity or parent feels is balanced. The celebrity's job is to be fit and your parent is at a different life stage. What matters is that you find your middle — the zone that enables you to thrive rather than simply survive. You learn how to appropriately respond. (Note the word *learn*. Again, I've purposely chosen an active word. You have to teach yourself to have appropriate responses.)

Appropriate responses are productive. Too often our health responses are the opposite of productive; they are disproportionate, all-or-nothing knee-jerk reactions. I get that this is easier said than done. Let's say you gain five pounds and are distressed by it. One unproductive, unmeasured response is, "I am worthless and fat and I will starve myself to lose this weight." On the other end of the spectrum the unproductive thought is, "Screw it! I gained five pounds; I might as well gain another five. Five pounds doesn't mean anything."

"Productive" — the 360 Interpretation!

· · · · · · · · · ·

Don't misunderstand my obsession with the word "productive" as an obsession with motion and action. I value silence and stillness and absolutely believe there is capacity for productivity available in both. I define "productivity" as any action (and stillness is action), conversation, or internal dialogue that will create (or move me towards) my desired result, feeling, or mindset. If the result I want is a better relationship with someone I care about (myself included), what is often most productive is silence and/or listening. Or, if the result I want is my body to recover, then sleeping or resting can be productive.

Instead, the problem needs to be given an appropriate response — a productive response — a response that will make your future self healthier. In the above example say, "Despite the five pounds I am still a worthwhile person. I love myself enough not to overreact but to take the rational steps needed so that in four weeks I will have lost the weight." Or as I say to my clients, be productive. Don't choose denial, but also don't lean in to depression. Find your equilibrium — your hammock. For you, maybe a productive response to gaining five pounds means cutting out your evening snack and adding in a few extra steps each day. For someone else, equilibrium might mean taking up a sport that they used to love and cutting sugar from their coffee. If the strategy you try doesn't work, have another measured response; don't dig deeper into a method that isn't working, but don't give up on health altogether. Instead of digging deeper or abandoning the dig, dig smarter. Learn from your experiences so that you can make smarter and more productive choices in the future.

To frame appropriate responses in a sillier way, understand making a less-than-ideal health choice as being served cold soup. If your soup is cold (you make a less-than-ideal choice) you should absolutely tell your server it is cold (being honest is an appropriate response), but don't punch the server in the face (the metaphorical equivalent of flogging yourself with belittling self-talk or punishing yourself through starvation).

SELF-TRUST, COMPASSION, AND APPROPRIATE RESPONSES

Self-trust is the internal belief that even if you have a health wobble — consume a cookie, skip a workout, or, for me, have a Fudgsicle — you will learn from the decision and course correct as quickly as possible. When you have trust in yourself, a mistake or a choice to indulge doesn't trigger cruel belittling self-talk or a negative health spiral of a food binge or an entire week of missed workouts. When you have self-trust, you use self-compassionate and productive self-talk to stay or get back on the horse.

Don't misunderstand me, though. Self-compassion is not a synonym for self-indulgence! Compassion has its roots in caring; care enough about yourself to make healthy choices. Think enough of yourself to expect yourself to try. Hold yourself to high standards because you love yourself. Don't justify skipping the gym or eating cake with, "Well, Kathleen told me to be compassionate." (Skipping the gym or eating junk is *not* compassion. Going to the gym and eating well are two key ways to show your body love.)

Your internal dialogue should be accurate, honest, and well-intentioned — based on helping yourself not hurting or belittling yourself. Your tone should be firm, passionate, and rigorous — just not belittling or harsh. Your thoughts and words should be beneficial, useful, and timely. Anxiety (future-thinking phantom thoughts) and loops of the past are not timely or useful. Harness what you can do in the current moment to benefit your situation and mood. Let go of thoughts that feed feelings of anger, self-doubt, and resentment.

An example of compassionate self-talk would be, "Self, that was not the most ideal choice. How can I make a better one next time?" versus "You are such a lazy ass; you can't do anything. No wonder no one loves you." Negative shame-filled self-talk does not put me in the mood to course correct and, in that moment, make the best choice possible. Cruel talk sets you up for failure — it inspires a negative health spiral.

By noting the issue with compassion and self-trust, you water the grounds for an appropriate response — you create an opportunity for your next choice to be positive and healthy. When I have a health wobble I try to say, "Kathleen, what would be the single thing I could do at this moment that would result in a future healthier and happier me?" When I frame it that way, I usually put down the second fudge bar.

As I already mentioned, for me, appropriate and moderate responses have typically been almost impossible. I am proud to announce this trend is turning. I am slowly becoming more secure and thus more secure in my decisions. I credit years of therapy and self-work. That said, I still find living by blanket rules easy and situational decisions fairly terrifying. Once I make a rule I never break it. I love rules. I don't have to think in the moment — I just follow the rule. I don't question if I should exercise — I just do. I don't question if I

Be the Boss of Your Own Health Company

• • • • • • • • • •

Reframe "work" and any related goals. Contrary to popular belief, work is not always pejorative — it is not always something negative or an action we have to do. By now you know my thoughts on the "have to–ness" of anything; it can feel suffocating and will inevitably invite your inner rebel to join the party.

So, reframe the work related to your physical and psychological health. It is not a job the boss is forcing on you. It is a job that you as the sole owner of your company — your body — are choosing to do!

One of the reasons I love my life, my job, and taking care of my health is that I decide what is best for all three. I am my own boss — in all respects.

---

should eat bread at a restaurant — I just say no. I don't question if I should put cream in my coffee — I don't use cream. It feels like I've been given the answers to the test. I don't even have to read the questions — I just rattle off memorized answers. I love the "I know the answer!" feeling. Strict lines in the sand are simple — for better or worse they quench any internal debate or questioning. I am uncomfortable with the feeling of "should I or shouldn't I?" Having to muddle through what choice to make is too time-consuming and opens Pandora's box. Yuck. Who needs it?

In theory, dedication, discipline, and habit formation are good qualities, but in practice I am beginning to realize that, although as a coping mechanism rules have served me well in many ways, it is the manifestation of a lack of self-trust. Don't get me wrong. I am not knocking myself. Living by non-negotiable rules was a critical element in my evolution from unhealthy teenager to healthy, active adult; rules were a critical first step. I am proud of my dedication and discipline.

I am not saying I want to throw in the towel and eat all the cake and not care about my choices. That is not only a cop-out but the polar extreme. What I am saying is, I don't want to have to bypass the problem-solving, rational aspect of making health choices. The "have to–ness" is what I have a problem with. I don't mind if I never eat many of my current non-negotiable foods, but I want to forgo consuming foods I don't like *not* because desserts are a non-negotiable no, but because I trust myself to make decisions that will make my future self happier — even when not governed by a rule. For example, I pretty much hate fruit-flavoured desserts, thus I am happy to never consume them again, but I don't want abstinence to be a non-negotiable. I want to trust myself enough to know that when a fruit dessert is offered I will think, I don't love that food. Eating it is so not worth it to me. Therefore, I'm going to pass.

My new-found understanding of the interconnectedness of trust and the ability to respond with compassion and intelligence (i.e., appropriate responses) came from reading John Gottman's book *The Science of Trust: Building Emotional Attunement for Couples*. Gottman explains the chicken-and-egg relationship between "happy couples," a "positive absorbing state," and "trust" between the partners. He maintains that happy couples in a "positive absorbing state" have a harder time "going negative." They stay in "negative" spaces

for shorter durations and have an easier time "getting back to the positive" — being "happy and emotionally connected" is their absorbing state that pulls them in like positive quicksand. Couples in a positive absorbing state can be compassionate with each other, look to the future not the past, and have measured, rational — not catastrophic — responses.

Couples are more likely to have a "positively absorbing state" if they trust each other. Why? One partner can only have a gracious interpretation of the other's actions, be empathetic, and be compassionate — and thus rationally work through the problem and "go positive" faster — when they trust their person. The more trust, the stronger the positive absorbing state. Put in Kathleen-speak: more often than not both partners have appropriate responses. Because they trust each other.

Your relationship with yourself — your self-talk and internal dialogue — is just that, a relationship. Thus, for you to be able to have appropriate responses with yourself you need self-trust; you need to be in a positively absorbing state with yourself! Your health choices cannot be divorced from your greater sense of self. The more you trust in you — your ability to make informed, rational decisions — the less often you will shame spiral and the more you will be able to make decisions not because you should or because it is a rule, but because you know your current and future self will be happier if you do. Trust will allow for rational thought and responses; it will foster the strength to dispute your inner critique and is aligned with self-compassion and empathy.

That last paragraph is key. Health is a process. You will fall off your horse, and when you do you need to be in a positive relationship with yourself — you need to be able to respond appropriately and have the trust to dust yourself off and get back on. Instead of "I am such a loser; I might as well quit now and eat more cookies" or "I love myself no matter what; might as well eat another cookie," you have to have the compassion and trust to say, "Yes, I had a cookie, and now I care enough about myself to go for a walk. As I walk I am going to decide if I enjoyed the cookie or if it wasn't worth it. If I enjoyed it — great. If it was an example of mindless eating, how do I ensure my future self doesn't make that choice again?" Think of it as living with an ever-present roommate in your head. Treat the roommate with respect so that you can build a trusting, productive relationship.

I have not fully worked through my relationship with self-trust — but that is okay.

I trust myself more than I did five years ago. Yay me for trending positive! But the journey is far from over, which is exciting; evolving and working is part of the joy of life.

So how do you cultivate the skills of self-trust, compassion, and the ability to respond rather than react? You embrace that self-compassion, self-trust, and appropriate responses are all skills that need to be learned through repetition. Health is a journey and learning these skills will take time. Think of all three as muscles. Muscles get stronger with use, so use them!

Keep going. Keep putting one foot in front of the other — in an atmosphere of growth (obviously), with an ear toward finding joy and potentially taking meditation skills off the mat. Curious what it means to take meditation off the mat? More on meditation coming up — I love a little anticipation!

 Consider starting a journal to keep track of your progress. Each night right down two instances when you did not exhibit appropriate responses, self-trust, or compassion. Then write out how the experience would have gone differently if you had — what would you have said, done, or thought differently.

FIND THE FUN

· ·

It is extremely demotivating to always do things because we have to or, even worse, because we feel the healthy choice is an appropriate punishment for ourselves. Additionally, who has the energy to make healthy choices when living a sad, joyless life? Of course you are going to want to rebel and eat cake or stay up late if everyday life feels like a series of obligations. I remember a conversation with my therapist, Dr. Pedder. I was frustrated by my inability to stop nighttime eating. I confessed that as I sat at my desk working, I constantly stopped to snack. She looked at me as if I were crazy and then said, very kindly, something like, "Well, of course you want to eat. The option you give yourself is working. Maybe instead of focusing on killing the eating habit, we need to work on finding you things to do other than working. Could you sleep? See friends? Read a book? Find a way to have fun?" Since then I have been actively trying to find the fun (hence my favourite hashtag, #FindingPocketsOfJoy). When I can't find any, I actively make some.

Too often people — the old Kathleen included — understand fun and joy as the opposite of adult obligations like working out and working; this polarization sets us up for failure. In *The Gifts of Imperfection*, Brené Brown says, "The opposite of play is not rest. The opposite of play is depression." In Kathleen-speak that equates to fun and joy don't happen only after chores — fun and joy are like breathing; they exist knitted into the fabric of everything. The more pockets of joy you can find, both at work and while working out, the happier, more energized, and more fulfilled you will be — and the more likely you will be to make healthy choices.

I often ask clients what their three Fs of the week are. The three Fs are fun, fitness, and food choices. Their fun is not something I want to hear about after I hear about their nutrition choices — fun is integral to making any and all healthy choices stick. Fun can be lounging poolside with friends or doing an activity you enjoy — but if you don't find ways to create joy in your life you will feel depressed and unmotivated; it is so much harder to make yourself move when you are depressed. Often, we think of mind, body, and spirit as being the cornerstones of a healthy lifestyle; in my opinion if you lose the joy, why bother with the others?

Let's connect this back up to a "positively absorbing state" and trust. This is key. The easier it is for you to absorb into the positives, the less likely you will be to numb your emotions with food and inactivity. Joy breeds joy. Joy breeds healthy choices. The more often you move and choose healthy alternatives, the more self-trust will flourish, and the easier it will be for you to make another healthy choice in the future. The cycle is self-perpetuating. Find every joy-filled little win you can; you never know which little win will initiate your forward positive spiral.

I often finish a client session by saying, "Find your kiwi."

This approach stemmed from a conversation I had with a client. She was no longer motivated to stick to her plan because eating healthy and exercising had become just another thing on her to-do list. When I asked her what healthy foods and modes of exercise she actually liked, she couldn't tell me. No wonder she was demotivated! She had unconsciously framed every healthy choice as a punishment. Her homework was to come up with two healthy things that

I am not suggesting you should love every moment of life or exercise — that is an unrealistic ask. Feel your emotions. I absolutely have sad moments. But instead of letting negatives bleed into the rest of your life, let your moments of joy snowball; then use the positive energy to lace up your shoes and get out the door.

she genuinely would be excited to eat or do. She decided she enjoyed kiwis (but never bought them because her family didn't like them) and gardening. I told her that whenever she wanted junk food she should instead have a kiwi (or another healthy choice worthy of the title of kiwi), and whenever she couldn't motivate herself to go to the gym that she should garden instead. That way she wouldn't feel constrained or deprived.

In light of that, a kiwi is something healthy that you truly love — or at least that you don't despise; we are always more apt to continue a program when it includes foods and activities one likes. Finding

We often need the things we find the hardest to make happen. When I am in a good mood, I give myself the okay to skip a workout. On days I am in a bad mood, I make exercise non-negotiable. I know I need it.

your kiwis is about gradually learning to associate making healthier choices with positive feelings. Put together two kiwi lists. Fill the first list with nutritionally dense, yummy food options. Make the second list exercise kiwis — activities that don't feel like a chore, like going on a bike adventure with your kids, dancing around the living room, walking the dog, or gardening. Instead of feeling sorry for yourself because you have to eat well or work out, ask yourself, Which of my yummy kiwis am I lucky enough to eat or do today?

MEDITATION

. . . .

I think of meditation as an awareness tool; a way to become an objective observer of your own thoughts, with the goal of decoupling from unproductive thought loops and attachments. Meditation breeds awareness, which opens the door for change — until you are aware of something (a thought, an action, an emotion) you can't consciously change it. To paraphrase Sharon Salzberg in *Real Happiness*, "The goal is not to become better at meditation, the goal is to become better at life." Or as Salzberg discussed on *The Tim Ferriss Show*, you can't

fail at meditation because the goal is not to control what is happening — in other words, to make your mind blank. The goal is to better understand and relate to what is happening in your body — thoughts, emotions, sensations — as you meditate.

There is a common — often fear-based — misconception that you have to be a particular type of person to meditate. The feeling that "I can't get my mind to shut up — I would be the worst at meditation" is all too common. If you can hear yourself uttering words like this, run — don't walk — *toward* a meditation practice. Typically, the more impossible meditation feels, the greater the body's need.

The intimidation factor is due, in large part, to the popular misunderstanding that the goal of meditation is to clear the mind completely — an unrealistic ask. The goal is to foster a better relationship with your thoughts. Success is not the lack of thoughts, but the ability to catch yourself and bring yourself back to the moment — back to the breath. Remember the metaphor of the swivel chair we used in chapter 4. When you are lost in meditation (lost in breath), the chair is stable. Swivelling is "wandering in thought"— letting your monkey mind take over. The mission is not to never swivel — we know that is unrealistic. The mission is to recognize you are swiveling as early as possible and with compassion pull yourself back to centre.

Let's circle back to trust. Here is the key point: The more self-trust developed, the quieter the monkey mind. When you trust that you will be able to intelligently come back to centre, the journey back will be less intense and shame-filled.

I love meditation because it is both a mirror and a model. Your dialogue during meditation will mirror your lack of self-trust. The techniques used during practice will then model how to act when those thoughts take over during life. Meditation mirrors how you think in life. Is your meditation full of catastrophic what-ifs or debilitating self-criticism? It is also a model for life; while mediating you learn how to breathe through and let go of your particular brand of brain propaganda and toxic thoughts. The aim is to translate the coping mechanism into life — for your practice to jump off the mat. Understand the difference between thinking and being a prisoner of your thoughts; let go of the unproductive never-ending to-do list, the pointless worry, the self-doubt, and the judgment. Change the relationship between you and

> You have no absolute power over the end product of anything, so make the process something you enjoy. If you can't enjoy it, make your responses ones you will respect. When it comes to meditation, this means stop trying to be the best at meditation, or even trying to make yourself love meditation, and just do it, consistently and with integrity.

your thoughts. Learn how to respond (in part a by-product of self-trust) rather than emotionally react (reacting almost always involves emotional extremes).

Thoughts — when appropriate — are vital to survival. Inappropriate, unproductive thoughts are not helpful. If you are being chased by a tiger, by all means activate that stress response as quickly as possible. But if your stress is because you are overwhelmed at work — and that stress typically causes you to binge eat — use meditation to gain perspective.

 Consider a 21-day meditation challenge. For 21 days, couple meditation with something you enjoy. For example, for 21 days take a bubble bath after you meditate. I have a hard time fitting in both yoga and meditation — but know I need both — so I recently challenged myself to 21 days of 22 minutes of yoga and 8 minutes of meditation a day. At the end of 21 days I felt accomplished, more centred, and more mobile.

Meditation also involves embracing another concept: thoughts are not facts. You are not your unhealthy, unproductive, sad, or angry thoughts or cravings. You can feel something and choose not to act on that feeling. Thoughts and emotions are always fleeting — simply visiting. With breath, we can let thoughts go. The breath is powerful. Breath signals the nervous system to switch from the sympathetic system (the stress response) to the parasympathetic system. The positives attributed to the parasympathetic nervous system include facilitating digestion, improving immune health, quieting the "monkey mind," and aiding restful sleep. The more often you let thoughts "go" — you don't act — the more self-trust is created. Your future self will be able to make future healthier choices with greater ease. To quote Rainer Maria Rilke in his poem "Go to the Limits of Your Longing," "Just keep going. No feeling is final."* I get the quote was not originally intended as a health beacon, but if it works it works.

This "thoughts are not facts" tenet has positively impacted all my relationships. When I perceive that my partner, James, has done something hurtful, I simply say, "Kathleen, your perception of the incident is not fact. Just talk to him." Or, when I feel there is "no way" I can make it through my

---

* *Rilke's Book of Hours: Love Poems to God* (New York: Riverhead Books, 2005).

day unless I eat copious amounts of sugar, I say, "Kathleen, thoughts are transitory. These negative thoughts have rented space in your body; they have not bought the property. You will feel better if you work without eating sugar, and even if you don't feel better, anyone can do anything for a day." I always feel better once I'm lost in work. Or I might take my therapist's advice and find the fun.

I found the idea that finally made me willing to brave meditation in Sharon Salzberg's book *Real Happiness*: "If you can breathe, you can meditate." I can breathe, so I thought, *Kathleen, lean in. Be curious. What is the worst that can happen?* It turns out I like meditation; it calms the never-ending to-do list in my head and siphons off daily me time. It keeps me centred between therapy sessions. It gives me a place to go when I feel overwhelmed and on the brink of making an inappropriate knee-jerk health choice. For example, I love cookie dough Quest bars — a non-food food that future Kathleen absolutely never feels good about having consumed. In the past when I would get anxious or overwhelmed I would say, "Screw it. This bar is better than nothing and will make me happy." Now I pause and take a few deep breaths. I am more able — most of the time — to say, "Kathleen, you

will feel better if you buy the hard-boiled egg from Starbucks or pop into a grocery store for a few vegetables."

Now, the caveat. I like my version of meditation. As I am sure you're aware by now, my philosophy for adopting any new habit is to learn the pros and cons, adopt what works for you, and ditch what doesn't. My meditation mix: a ten-minute personalized practice (someone else's voice is a deterrent) within an atmosphere of growth. Much of what I always appreciate is the philosophy behind a practice — the why.

In terms of meditation, that means that if you're curious, experiment. Find a class, teacher, or personal practice you can relate to. Try breathing meditation, sound meditation, loving kindness meditation, or maybe a mindfulness meditation. Meditate in the morning to frame your day, during lunch to centre yourself, or at night as part of a bedtime ritual. Maybe your meditation mix is simply committing to taking ten deep breaths whenever you are stressed. Maybe it's using an app such as Headspace.

There are no miracle solutions. Take meditation for what it is: one component of your overall health recipe, assuming it works for you!

Yes, the parasympathetic nervous system facilitates a state in which healing is better able to occur, but meditation should not replace other forms of health care. To quote my colleague Harry, "Breathing is always good, but breathing will not eliminate my meniscus tear."

Or related more specifically to this chapter, meditating for a month will not automatically imbue you with self-trust or the ability to have instant fun. Meditation is a practice. Building self-trust takes time. Learning to have appropriate responses is one of the wonderful problems of the privilege of being alive. We are human. We are gifted with the ability to learn and grow. Good things take work. As Tom Hanks says in *A League of Their Own*, "It's supposed to be hard. The hard is what makes it great." I am not sure if something has to be hard to be great (I am still thinking on that), but I do know that adopting a healthier lifestyle and mindset is hard — and that it is also worthwhile, so I am totally okay with the work entailed.

Also, keep in mind that, like everything, meditation only works if you work it; meditation will not aid weight loss if you're eating five muffins a day and it will not build self-trust if you make a wish not a goal to meditate and don't follow through.

I CHALLENGE YOU TO FAIL

Create a positive absorbing state with yourself — make sure the roommate in your head is friendly — so that when you fumble or completely fall off your horse you can do so within an atmosphere of growth, with an ability to respond rather than react and thus course correct as quickly as possible.

Most of us have an enemy living inside our heads. We are extremely cruel to ourselves. (Reflect on this for a minute. The fact that we spend the majority of our day with someone who is being mean to us — not believing in us — is heartbreaking. No wonder so many of us overeat, drink too much, and under-exercise!) Internally, we use a belittling tone of voice and rude language that we would never use on the barista at Starbucks — let alone a loved one!

The golden rule has to go both ways; yes, do unto others as you would want others to

> Build your personal health literacy. Learn about you — your health triggers, what works, and what doesn't. Health literacy is a process. Aim to continue learning and growing. Meditation, journaling, and self-reflection are all helpful ways to build literacy.

do unto you, but also do unto yourself as you would do unto others. Learn to have empathy and compassion for yourself and create a positive internal state. Learn to be on your own side. (I am lecturing myself here … my inner voice is not always kind. I am working on her, but it is a process.)

As you work to create your positive internal state, know you will fail — falling is part of the process — but make sure you are failing versus simply not trying, and fall with the goal of trending positive. Gradually aim to make your falls less severe and your course corrections more immediate.

As Hillary Clinton said in her book *What Happened*, "Get caught trying."* Don't procrastinate starting your health

_____
* Hillary Rodham Clinton, *What Happened* (New York: Simon & Schuster, 2017).

journey because of a fear of failure. Your process doesn't have to be perfect — perfect is not possible. Your process just has to start. Yes, adopting a healthier lifestyle and fostering a positive relationship with yourself — building trust — is not simple or easy, but as I often tell clients, working is winning. Tell yourself, "The only thing not allowed is giving up."

Experiment. Work to find your kiwis. Work to understand your emotions — journal or consider therapy. Try meditation. It has the potential to create a space where you can change your relationships with your thoughts so that off the mat you will have tools in your emotional toolbox to respond rather than react to stimuli — tools that allow you to reflect on your actions and thoughts, and thus make decisions your future self will be proud of.

Make an overarching goal to connect with your body. To, as my wonderful client Alexi says, replace simply having a body with *living* in *your* body. Too many of us have grown disconnected from our own bodies — we end up floating, almost as if in someone else's body. We don't know what our kiwis are, what gives us joy, what we love. I want my readers to learn to love, trust, and own their bodies rather than merely existing within them!

Turn Failure into Fodder

· · · · · · · · · ·

Live life like you are a comedian — always looking for a good story to tell.

Stop being afraid to fail or embarrassed if you falter or make an unhealthy choice. We all fail. The trick is to get back up and (with gusto, when possible) tell the story with humour. Failing is not something to have shame about and keep to yourself; when you hide a story, you give it power.

Tell the world how mightily you failed and then *show* the world how you got up and learned from that failure.

Establish a goal to be on your own side. Embrace that health — like life — is a process. Become aware of your choices — the tone of your self-talk being a choice — and learn and grow through your experiences. Always rigorously analyze any act (missed workout, negative self-talk, food binge, et cetera), but do not connect the act to your worth as a human being. Always address the incident rather than attacking your character. If you fall off your health horse (you're mean to yourself, you shame yourself, you over-indulge), walk yourself firmly — yet kindly and with compassion — through the experience. Note your emotions and figure out why the situation triggered you. Reverting back is not a failure; it is an opportunity to figure out *why*, in that moment, you could not be your own best friend.

Work with yourself to practise self-trust, self-compassion, and appropriate responses so that you have a supportive companion to take with you on your health journey.

I know you can do it. Put one foot in front of the other. Take your next best step. Start!

> Stop trying to live your life to impress an invisible jury. All that matters is that you are proud of your own choices. Be authentic. Live with integrity.

Final Musings

Congratulations on reaching the end of the book! You now have everything you need to create — yes, that active word again — your fittest (and happiest, most productive) future self.

- You have the tools to curate your own health — the tools to consume any diet, workout, or mindset information and parse out the relative data to your individualized NUTRITIONmix, WORKOUTmix, and MINDSETmix.

- You have the capacity to sift through any health information and latch on to the pros — relative to your goals and genetics — and discard options with too many cons.

- You have the tools to be an intelligent mix maker — to do you!

- You have the wherewithal to know that your fittest self cannot be found. Long-term success is created within you!

The world is your oyster. Your health journey starts *now*!

TEN THINGS I KNOW FOR SURE

• •

Your health journey may start now, but keep in mind that health is a process and as such will — and must — evolve. My own journey has been anything but linear, and it started almost twenty years ago, but it has been unbelievably fruitful. I was a chubby, awkward adolescent. I hated being active. I hated my body. I hated myself. Now I love being active and (mostly) feel confident in my own skin. Throughout my journey I have cried many times. I have wanted to give up too many times to count. But I didn't.

After almost twenty years in the fitness field I have learned this for certain: the key is to always keep going, to never give up. To never shy away from hard work. To give fear the finger!

There are a few other things I know for sure — concepts I consider my guiding principles. I offer them to you to use as a jumping off point. Feel free to borrow them until you form your own list.

1. HEALTH IS AN INSIDE JOB. YOU CAN'T BUY IT. YOU CAN'T FORCE SOMEONE ELSE TO CREATE IT FOR THEMSELVES OR FOR YOU. YOU HAVE TO OWN YOUR HEALTH CHOICES.

Lots of people can support your journey. I believe it takes a village. You can enlist a fitness buddy, find a motivational running group, or even enlist a therapist, but ultimately *you* have to do the work. You need to use help in a productive way, and you have to use the help to form a version of yourself that you respect. In her TED Talk, Anne Lamott says, "Nothing outside of you will help in any lasting way, except if you're waiting for an organ." Achieving your perfect weight will not make you happy unless you are actually happy with yourself first. Buying the best gym clothes or having the fanciest trainer won't buy a fit body — or happiness or motivation. External objects can never replace productive self-talk and a positive — or at least a trending positive — relationship with self.

2. **YOU NEED TO LOVE YOURSELF. HECK, START WITH AT *LEAST* LIKING YOURSELF, EVEN MILDLY.**

Your thoughts are not only key, but they are up to you. Your personal health narrative — your internal version of who you are and what you are capable of — are chosen by you. If your narrative is not working for you, choose a new one. As Gandhi said, "Beliefs become thoughts. Thoughts become words. Words become actions. Actions become habits. Habits become values. Values become destiny." In Kathleen-speak, thinking about becoming healthier is obviously not enough; thoughts are not everything, but thoughts start the process. If your narrative is not working for you, choose a new one. Dig deep. Find the game-changing narrative. Choose the thoughts that open up the possibility of taking you down the road to beautiful health.

3. **IT'S IMPORTANT TO DECIDE WHOSE OPINIONS AND VALUES MATTER TO YOU.**

Let go of the need to be liked by everyone. You don't like everyone and not everyone is going to like you or approve of your actions, and that is okay. You are not a politician. Decide who the few people in your life are that you respect. Care what they think. Decide on your values. Care about people who share the same values. Let go of useless noise. Stop feeling your self-worth balloon be deflated by a lack of social media attention.

Create your life map — a program that works for you and respects who *you* are. Decide what you want to achieve and who you want to be. Do you. If you're not sure who you are, decide who you don't want to be — who you are not — and lean away from that.

4. **SELF-CARE IS NOT SELFISH; YOU CAN'T EXHALE IF YOU DON'T INHALE!**

You can't be of any service to anyone — including yourself — if you're dead, burned out, exhausted, et cetera. You can't exhale if you don't inhale!

Inhaling includes activities that refuel you, activities that fill you with energy, that allow you to be still and recharge, that make you feel like the most centred, authentic version of you. For me these include running, sleeping, meditation, and listening to audiobooks. Others might inhale through painting, walking, or gardening.

You exhale by doing activities for others and by being a productive member of society; think fulfilling obligations, being an outstanding parent or employee, or grinding through everyday adult tasks. Too many of us prioritize these exhaling activities at the expense of our own health; acts of self-care are framed as, at best, nice when time permits and, more commonly, as a complex cocktail of self-indulgence, selfishness, and narcissism.

Being active and taking the time to eat well — acts of self-care — are not selfish! In fact, acts of self-care enable you to create the healthy, productive, emotionally intelligent, and happiest future self that you (and your loved ones and co-workers) want and require you to be. It's not about always prioritizing inhaling over exhaling. But too many of us exhale at the expense of ourselves; you can't produce the best version of you if you constantly prioritize exhale activities at the expense of inhaling needs.

Exhaling — being productive and busy — is not inherently bad; it is all a matter of degrees. As Brené Brown says in *The Gifts of Imperfection*, being "too busy" is not a badge of honour. Being too busy means you are out of balance. Creating a healthier mind and body comes through giving to yourself and giving to others. If you bias toward inhaling, add exhale activities to your life. If you only exhale — typically exhalers have nebulous boundaries — take time to inhale.

5. **ON THE INSIDE, EVERYONE IS SCARED, FLAWED, AND BROKEN. EVEN PEOPLE WHO SEEM TO HAVE IT ALL FIGURED OUT DON'T.**

Embrace that we are all human and that we are all flawed. So get moving in all of your flaws. Don't let the fear of others being better than you stop you from bettering yourself. Give fear the finger. As we discussed in chapter 5, think of fear as "false evidence appearing real." We fear others have it all figured out and we don't, so we don't go for the walk or we don't go to the gym or we don't try for a new job. Ask yourself what you can do to limit interference and increase possibilities. When you are afraid, tell yourself that fear means "face everything and rise." Let go of perfectionism. Let go of the desire to be perfect. Perfect is not possible. No one is perfect. Perfectionism simply becomes a method of self-sabotage — a way to stay stuck and to be unproductive and ultimately self-destructive. Stay in your own lane.

6. YOU NEED TO STOP EXPENDING ENERGY THINKING ABOUT WHAT OTHERS ARE DOING AND SAYING. USE YOUR ENERGY ON YOU.

I am obviously not arguing that you should stop being a parent or being a good partner or being a good person and thinking of others. But the only person you have direct control over is yourself. Get *yourself* together. Don't think about the food and exercise choices that your friend is making. Stop trying to help someone be fitter. If they ask, sure, add helpful thoughts, but their health journey is theirs. As Anne Lamott says in her TED Talk, "Help is the sunny side of control." Stop helping — unless

asked. Focus your attention on your journey. If you want to control someone, control you.

7. GRIT AND PERSEVERANCE ARE KEY. WHEN YOU FALL, GET UP AND LEARN.

We all fall. Falling is part of being human. Falling can either destroy you or the experiences can make you stronger. Don't ignore misdoings or justify hurting others by stating it was a fall — obviously wrongdoings are wrongdoings. I am not giving you the okay to be an ass — but use every situation as information. Have grit. Persevere. Learn. Grow. When I was diagnosed with dyslexia I could have decided to ditch my love of writing. I didn't. I used it as motivation to get better. I used it as motivation to always have a great editor. My friend and colleague Kathryn reads all my work. I truly believe she makes my work better — and that many writers could benefit from a little bit of enforced editing. As Hillary Clinton wrote in her book *What Happened*, the question is not if you are flawed or if you make mistakes; it is "What do you do about your flaws?" Do you learn from your mistakes so you can do and be better in the future? Or do you reject the hard work of self-improvement? To use Kathleen-speak, when you fall off your horse, do you use it as an excuse to eat another cookie or do you learn from the fall and get back on your horse as a more informed rider? Stop trying to find short cuts. Good things — more often than not — take time.

8. THE ONLY MOMENT YOU HAVE TRUE CONTROL OVER IS NOW.

Sure, actions today will affect the future, but not if you don't actually act today. As Jon Kabat-Zinn wrote in *Wherever You Go, There You Are*, "Whatever has happened to you, it has already happened. The important question is, how are you going to handle it?" He asks his readers to ponder the important question, Now what? In Kathleen-speak, this moment is really all we have to work with. Stop talking about what you are going to do and just do it. Reflect on what you value, then do it now — not tomorrow. You can't control the past, and the only way to influence the future is through this moment. So pause — then act in this moment the way you want your future self to act. In the

pause, lean away from negative brain propaganda; lean toward the actions you want your future self to take.

Remember, too, that inaction is also action. Often it feels like by doing nothing you are safe, but not changing is an active choice. You are acting as you have always done, deepening your "stuckness."

9. HEALTH HAPPENS MOMENT BY MOMENT, BIT BY BIT. THE SECRET TO LIFE AND HEALTH IS BUM IN THE SEAT TIME AND JUST STARTING!

Health takes practice. Your unhealthy habits were not formed in a day. It is unrealistic to think your healthier habits will be formed in a day. Devote yourself to lots of time practising your new lifestyle. You cannot become your fitter future self overnight.

The hardest part of anything is often just starting. So don't get caught in the health weeds. Too much analysis is paralysis. The techniques in this book will be helpful, but in the end you have to start. Once you start an activity program — even if it is simply to walk — you can always tweak or add to the program, but if you never start, you have nothing to tweak. Something is always better than nothing and you have to start somewhere.

Conditions will never be perfect. Just go. Once you've done one workout, it will be physically and psychologically easier to do another and another and another. Before you know it you will be on your way to your version of fit.

10. THE WORSE YOUR DAY, THE MORE IMPORTANT THE WORKOUT.

Don't wait for the best day or moment to work out. Working out will make you feel better. Being active will make you more functional and give you a sense of control. Embrace the truism that life is not perfect and shitty days and moments are inevitable — not in a "poor me" way, but in a way that says this day might be dramatically imperfect, but that doesn't give me a justification to be inactive or make unhealthy decisions. In her TED Talk, Anne Lamott describes life as a "mixed grill of happy anticipation and dread." In Kathleen-speak that means the fitter you are, the more coping mechanisms and strength you will have to survive the ups and downs of a day.

TIPS FOR YOUR NEXT STEPS

You have the information and the tools needed to create your mixes. Now the hard part begins … or continues … or ends. I am never sure which part of the health process is the hardest — the before, during, or after a health awakening.

Being an unhealthy, unhappy teenager was excruciatingly hard, but I was almost too unaware to own my deep sorrow and the inherent hardness of every day. I ate my sorrow down into myself. Now, in some ways every moment is harder because I have embraced that each moment is the only moment I have direct control over. Every moment and every day is a lesson and a journey. I am acutely aware of the privilege of learning that life offers, which in some ways is hard, but it is happy hard, it is productive hard; it is conscious, and it is fruitful.

As you begin or progress, embrace three things.

First, forming your mixes — and then sticking to them — requires a growth mindset! I wish I could tell you that your health journey will be simple and linear, that reading this book will keep you on your health horse forever. I won't say any of that. There is no quick fix for health. You will fall. I do every day. I fall, but my falls this month are smaller in scale than ten years ago, or even two years ago. And now I course correct faster and aim to learn from every deviation.

Make your goal to trend positive — to learn. In many ways I wish a few medium, non-destructive — let's call them *slips* — on you, because when you slip or fall in the muck, you have the opportunity to get up and learn from that fall. The fantastic — and often freeing — element of becoming an active mix maker is that (when used properly) an experience that previously would have thrown you off of your horse becomes fodder for growth and learning; instead of being paralyzing, failing becomes a launching ground for long-term success!

Think of life — which includes your health process — as a giant feedback loop.

Try something. If it works, great. Do it again. If it doesn't work, possibly even better; often something "not working" teaches you more than something going as planned. Learn from every experience. Make continually more informed — and more tailored to you and your "ness" — decisions each day.

Second, know that growth takes effort. The thing is, living even in a stuck state takes effort too; spinning your wheels in anxiety and useless thought is often more exhausting than doing something. No matter what, you can't jump over the effort piece — but you can jump over useless effort. Why spin your wheels to get nowhere? As Stephen R. Covey in *The 7 Habits of Highly Effective People* states, "Being busy is different than being productive"; don't confuse stressing about your health and criticizing other people's health choices (treading water — unproductive busy brain work) with taking positive steps to change your health (swimming forward). Furiously treading water may feel productive — and the positive is it keeps you from dying — but it doesn't get you to your end goal. You survive; you don't thrive. Treading water is the equivalent of busy work — it is not productive!

Every day is going to take effort, so make it productive effort. Instead of wasting time on belittling self-talk and self-sabotage, harness and make the best use of your energy, time, and intellect.

Third, know that in every moment lies a choice — you are always at a fork in the road. You can choose to make a compassionate, aware, responsive choice — however small — that will move your health journey on a positive trajectory. Or, you can choose to react to stimuli — to move toward what I often call *health shit creek*. I am not arguing making a productive choice will guarantee immediate success, but at least productive, aware choices give you the possibility of success. We move toward shit creek sometimes — small steps in that direction are to be expected — just simply try and note the choice as quickly as possible so you can course correct.

Don't simply read this book and forget about it. Use the text to keep you on your health horse — especially the various inspirational features. Reread the book as many times as necessary, and use the Kathleenisms, challenges, and personal stories as helping hands. Information is useless if you don't put it into action — the features are there to give you effective in the moment action steps. Try a new challenge each week. Put the Kathleenisms and other inspirations on sticky notes or in your phone — read them when you need motivation. Read my personal stories when you feel discouraged. Remind yourself that you are not alone. I have been there — I have felt your frustration. Think of my personal stories as a friendly, compassionate hug. Imagine me there saying, "I did it and I know you can as well."

YOUR FITTEST FUTURE SELF AWAITS

You can do this! The key is to act now!

I saw a sign at IKEA that said, "Your future is what you do today not what you do tomorrow." Ditch the quest to find the perfect anything. Instead, work to have sincere health intentions and clear principles.

Be honest with yourself. Curate your own WORKOUTmix, NUTRITIONmix, and MINDSETmix, but remember that your attitude and dedication to your health — and thus how you interpret rules — are what matter. Situations change, but the values and principles you use to navigate each situation need to stay constant.

Remember to embrace the pause. Work to respond and reflect rather than react.

Work to create a positive relationship with yourself — move toward healthy self-talk. Make yourself your own best friend.

Breathe. Grow. Have a critical beginners mind. Be curious. Listen — really listen — don't just listen until it is your turn to talk. Reflect. Learn. Persevere. Work to build grit. Embrace the importance of taking micro health steps; note all little wins.

Be the author of your own life story. Don't get caught up in someone else's story. Don't let what other people think of you slowly deflate your "ness" like air slowly seeping from a tire.

Adopting a healthier lifestyle can be frustrating, but the journey is ultimately an extremely rewarding, enriching, and worthwhile process. Through the frustration comes the opportunity for personal and interpersonal growth and development.

Most importantly, act. Stop talking about what you will do and *do*!

Kathleen's Recommendations for Growth, Learning, and Joy

The relationship I have with self-help and self development books (typically audiobooks) and podcasts is almost enigmatic. To say I love them doesn't cut it. To say they have been — and will continue to be — my master teachers gives the relationship some comprehensible form but is still not rich enough in description. I have been known to describe my various audio experiences as my therapy between therapy sessions and a way to consistently sharpen my emotional muscles — I am a believer in consistency. I often compare my emotional growth to my physical growth saying, "Just as you don't get physically fit in one day, you don't get emotionally fit in one therapy session a month. Going to my therapist is analogous to seeing a trainer once a month for a program. Reading and listening to references that challenge my brain is my daily dose of psychological fitness, analogous to my daily stretching or running routine."

Anyone who knows me knows that — for better or worse, since my quotes and mantras can be annoying — it is often hard to disentangle me from whatever book I am reading; I become momentarily enmeshed. If I find the information useful it then becomes woven into the fabric of both my life and fitness philosophy. The information is more than simply information to me — learning is an opportunity for growth, but also for joy. I love the act of learning and incorporating that new knowledge into my work and personal life.

Hence this list. While writing *Your Fittest Future Self* I — both personally and professionally — drew inspiration and information from many books, authors, and podcasts. I have compiled the key sources into this list, with the hope that they will inspire your growth as much as they've helped mine.

NUTRITION

• •

Acquista, Angelo. *The Mediterranean Prescription: Meal Plans and Recipes to Help You Stay Slim and Healthy for the Rest of Your Life* (New York: Ballentine Books, 2006). A good, comprehensive guide for exploring a Mediterranean diet.

Bean, Anita. *The Complete Guide to Sports Nutrition*, 7th edition (London: A&C Black, 2013). As an athlete — and a trainer working with active individuals — an excellent and comprehensive reference for nutrition information related to recovery, performance, activity, and longevity.

Beck, Judith S. *The Beck Diet Solution: Train Your Brain to Think Like a Thin Person* (New York: HarperCollins, 2015). I particularly found her image of only eating out of the top tier or two of the cake helpful, as I discussed in chapter 9.

Haas, Elson. *Staying Healthy with Nutrition: The Complete Guide to Diet and Nutritional Medicine* (Berkley: Celestial Arts, 2006). CSNN (Canadian School of Natural Nutrition) — the school I attended to become a nutritionist — uses this as one of its seminal texts; I found it an excellent — and comprehensive — reference guide for all things "nutrition."

Taubes, Gary. *Why We Get Fat and What to Do About It* (New York, Anchor Books, 2011). I appreciated Gary's book because it highlighted for me, once again, how complicated the human body is and why most health advice just doesn't work. I recommend Taubes' book to anyone wanting to more fully understand the interaction of genetics, sugar, and hormones in the human body.

FITNESS

· ·

Stanton, John. *Running: The Complete Guide to Building Your Running Program* (Toronto: Penguin Canada, 2010). This book helped me when I started running — a good basic reference text.

Trotter, Kathleen. *Finding Your Fit: A Compassionate Trainer's Guide to Making Fitness a Lifelong Habit* (Toronto: Dundurn, 2016). Of course I'm partial to this one! The four fitness personalities are explained in greater detail, and more workout ideas and motivational strategies are offered.

Trotter, Kathleen. *Huffington Post* blogs (huffingtonpost.ca/author/kathleen-trotter). In many ways I solidified my thoughts for *Your Fittest Future Self* through writing these blogs. Browse to get more workout ideas and strategies.

MINDSET

· ·

Brach, Tara. *Radical Acceptance: Embracing Your Life With the Heart of a Buddha* (New York: Bantam Bell, 2003). This book explores how Buddhist teachings can help us to heal feelings of not good enough.

Brown, Brené. *Braving the Wilderness: The Quest for True Belonging and the Courage to Stand Alone* (New York: Random House, 2017). This one is about true belonging.

Brown, Brené. *Daring Greatly: How the Courage to Be Vulnerable Transforms the Way We Live, Love, Parent, and Lead* (New York: Avery, 2015). This book reframes vulnerability as a pathway to courage and meaningful connection.

Brown, Brené. *The Gifts of Imperfection: Let Go of Who You Think You're Supposed to Be and Embrace Who You Are* (Center City: Hazelden Publishing, 2010). This book validated my bugaboo with perfection and articulated the importance of speaking your shame, that being too busy is not a badge of honour, and that joy is essential to the process of life and not something you have after you reach your goals.

Brown, Brené. *Rising Strong: How the Ability to Reset Transforms the Way We Live, Love, Parent, and Lead* (New York: Random House, 2017). I'm sure by now you know how important I think falling — and *learning* from falls — is. This book is about rising stronger after setbacks.

Chapman, Gary. *The Five Love Languages: The Secret to Love that Lasts* (Chicago: Northfield Publishing, 2015). This book articulated for me that we all have different ways (languages) of giving and receiving love (physical touch, gifts, acts of service, et cetera) and the importance of understanding your own love language, as well as the languages of those we care for.

Covey, Stephen R. *The 7 Habits of Highly Effective People: Powerful Lessons in Personal Change* (New York: Simon & Schuster, 2013). A classic. Traditionally a business book, but it offers practical approaches for personal change.

Duckworth, Angela. *Grit: The Power of Passion and Perseverance* (New York: Scribner, 2016). As you know, I believe perseverance is key. This details how success comes from grit not talent.

Duhigg, Charles. *The Power of Habit: Why We Do What We Do in Life and Business* (New York: Random House, 2012). As it sounds, this book is all about how habits work and how we can change them or use them to our advantage.

Duhigg, Charles. *Smarter Faster Better: The Transformative Power of Real Productivity* (New York: Random House, 2017). This book presents eight key productivity concepts, illustrated by examples from highly-productive people.

Dweck, Carol. *Mindset: The New Psychology of Success* (New York: Ballentine Books, 2007). This book gave me the language to delve deeper into what growth actually means and to explain the significance of growth.

Ferriss, Tim. *The 4-Hour Work Week: Escape 9–5, Live Anywhere, and Join the New Rich* (New York: Crown Publishers, 2009). This book teaches you how to work smarter not harder and to get more with less.

Gallwey, W. Timothy. *The Inner Game of Tennis: The Classic Guide to the Mental Side of Peak Performance* (New York, Random House, 1997). Another classic. This is about improving performance in any activity.

Gottman, John. *The Science of Trust: Building Emotional Attunement for Couples* (New York: W.W. Norton, 2011). This book was key to my understanding of a positive absorbing state and healthy relationships.

Hendrix, Harville. *Getting the Love You Want: A Guide for Couples* (New York: Henry

Holt, 2008). Another classic. This one tackles creating loving, supportive relationships.

Kabat-Zinn, Jon. *Wherever You Go, There You Are: Mindfulness Meditation in Everyday Life* (New York: Hachette Books, 2005). A classic on mindfulness meditation and mindfulness-based stress reduction.

Lamott, Anne. *12 Truths I Learned from Life and Writing* (TED Talk, 2017). This inspiration for the things I know for sure is about being human in this crazy world.

Lyubomirsky, Sonja. *The How of Happiness: A New Approach to Getting the Life You Want* (New York: Penguin Press, 2008). This is a practical approach to incorporating strategies for happiness into your life.

Manson, Mark. *The Subtle Art of Not Giving a F*ck: A Counterintuitive Approach to Living a Good Life* (New York: HarperCollins, 2016). This book looks at how overrated positivity is and uses honesty to avoid coddling and self-indulgence.

Marcus, Aubrey. *Own the Day, Own Your Life: Optimized Practices for Waking, Working, Learning, Eating, Training, Playing, Sleeping, and Sex* (New York, HarperCollins, 2018). This is next on my to-read list.

Mumford, George. *The Mindful Athlete: Secrets to Pure Performance* (Berkeley: Parallax Press, 2015). This is an exploration of the mind and how we all — athletes and regular Joe Blows — get in our own way physically and psychologically. His description of right effort was key for me.

Neff, Kristin. *Self-Compassion: The Proven Power of Being Kind to Yourself* (New York: HarperCollins, 2011). This was influential on my thinking about self-love and self-compassion.

Robbins, Tony. *Money: Master the Game — 7 Simple Steps to Financial Freedom* (New York: Simon & Schuster, 2014). Technically a finance book, but a must-read for personal development in general.

Robbins, Tony. *Unshakeable: Your Financial Freedom Playbook* (New York: Simon & Schuster, 2017). Another finance book with useful insights for personal development.

Rubin, Gretchen. *Better Than Before: Mastering the Habits of Our Everyday Lives* (Toronto: Anchor Canada, 2015). This book provides an analytical and scientific framework for our everyday habits, along with strategies to replace our less-than-ideal habits with healthier ones.

Rubin, Gretchen. *The Four Tendencies: The Indispensable Personality Profiles That Reveal How to Make Your Life Better (and Other People's Lives Better, Too)* (New York: Harmony, 2017). This book outlines four categories for how we tend to respond to expectations and suggests strategies to improve relationships tailored to how we approach life.

Rubin, Gretchen. *The Happiness Project* (New York: HarperCollins, 2012). This details her year-long quest to learn how to better enjoy and appreciate life.

Salzberg, Sharon. *Real Happiness: The Power of Meditation — A 28-Day Program* (New York: Workman Publishing, 2010). This book challenged the old Kathleen's resistance to meditation and convinced me to give it a try.

Seligman, Martin. *Authentic Happiness: Using the New Positive Psychology to Realize Your Potential for Lasting Fulfillment* (New York: Atria, 2013). This book helps you to identify your strengths and virtues and take full advantage of them.

PODCASTS

Bussin, Jamie. *The Tonic Podcast* (zoomerradio.ca/category/show/tonic/the-tonic-show-podcast/). A podcast about health and wellness.

Ferriss, Tim. *The Tim Ferriss Show* (tim.blog/podcast/). Long-form interviews with world-class performers from various walks of life with the goal of gleaning tactics, tools, and routines you can implement to improve your own life.

Fit Chicks Chat (fitchicksacademy.com/category/fit-chicks-podcast). The Fit Chicks Academy — run by two inspiring women, Laura Jackson and Amanda Quinn — offers bootcamps, nutrition programs, certifications, resources, and a podcast for women looking to live a healthier and "fierce" life. I appreciate Laura and Amanda's long-term, sustainable, and positive approach to health. Amanda interviewed me on episode 57 of their podcast. We discuss how small health changes add up, why it is important to frame making healthy choices as a privilege, and how to "own" your health journey so you can feel excited rather than overwhelmed.

Misner, Allan. *40+ Fitness Podcast* (40plusfitnesspodcast.com/podcast/). All about fitness after 40.

The Other F Word (theotherfwordpodcast.com). This is about taking the shame out of failure — I really respect the hosts and the message.

Acknowledgements

I consider myself an extremely lucky duck. I share my life with an almost innumerable cohort of outstanding individuals — people who not only make my life possible but also make my life worth living. One thing these people have taught me is that even if I could exist as an island, I would not want to. My village is a vital component of my happiness recipe. Everyone — from my unwaveringly supportive partner and family to my health care professionals — ensure that my life is both joyful and meaningful.

I will start by thanking my family — especially my exquisite mother and my best friend and partner, James — who make it clear daily that I am worthy of love. To paraphrase Kristin Neff in her book *Self-Compassion*, humans often aim high, desire success and achievement, get stuck on the hedonistic treadmill, reach for the stars, et cetera, in an attempt to find love. I am blessed that I can reach for the stars because I am curious about the stars — not because I'm looking for love. I have the privilege of knowing that my success is never a prerequisite. I know I am loved as me.

I won the mother lottery. My mom not only taught me how to love, she ingrained in me life coping skills and mottos, such as, In life, there is always a solution. This childhood lesson became one of the cornerstones of my fitness philosophy. My partner, James, makes my heart hurt with love — and often with laughter; he has been known to make me laugh so hard that I have to squeak out, "Stop talking ... can't breathe." My second family — Harriet, Clay, Emma, Kate, Best, Jane, and Esme — taught me to believe in something, to have opinions, and to stand tall in those opinions. My dad and sister offer friendship and support and always welcome me to Montreal with open arms. My godmother, Maureen, is a second mom and a wonderful friend and confidante. My sister deserves special kudos for — without fail — being willing to entertain my texts and phone calls — even at midnight on New Year's Eve. (Tris, I will be eternally grateful for that call.)

Next, I want to thank the people in the category of those I could *not* live without. First, Kathryn. Kathryn edits *all* of my work before *anyone* else sees it. I am highly dyslexic and having Kathryn gives me the gumption to share my writing with the world. I trust Kathryn implicitly; she is smart, kind, an awesome editor, and sort of my second brain. Next, Tracy Noonan. Tracy is the talented graphic designer behind my new website. Plus, Tracy handles all my day-to-day tech stuff. As everyone knows, I suck at tech. I love Tracy. Enough said. Next, the two doctors in my life. My therapist, Dr. Petter, and my naturopath, Dr. Kendall-Reed (or as I often call her, "Dr. Penny"). Dr. Penny turned my health around. Many don't know how sick I was a few years ago. At the time I didn't really talk about it. I am only now starting to open up about the experience. The net of it is that without Penny I would not have gotten back to the version of Kathleen I feel comfortable being. The final person in this category is my amazing friend Emily. Emily is the kind of friend who couriers you a care package for your birthday weekend away *and* quickly whips up mock-up book covers *and* has the capacity to inspire a book topic over pedicures. Yep, that is right, Em not only helped design the cover of *Your Fittest Future Self* but also helped me brainstorm the original concept. Thank you, Emily.

That leads nicely into a broad thank you to all my friends. Ever heard the aphorism "tell something bad to a friend and it becomes half as bad. Tell something good to a friend and it becomes doubly as good"? Well, that is how I feel about all of my friends. Thank you, Tari, Jenn and Noah, Krista, Leanne, Miriam, Tara, Ashik, Julie, Jack, Kristina,

Louise and Charles, Kate, Harry and Jessica, Josh and Megan, and Mellissa. Two special friend shout-outs: First, thank you to Julie and Ashik — I often feel I should pay you for your business consults and advice. Second, thank you to Harry for making *any* and *all* experiences fun, for being my "Trainer Chat" co-host, for being a friend who is also a colleague (and thus someone I can talk fitness with for hours without any eyes rolling), and for ensuring that the CanFitPro conference is a yearly awesome event. I am honoured to share the camera with Harry every Friday — Harry makes being on camera fun!

No acknowledgment section would be complete without a thank you to all of my amazing clients. I love my life in large part because I get to spend my days chatting with amazing people. Two special shout-outs: First to Ron who was my first client ever and who is still training with me. Second to Reva. Reva introduced me to Brené Brown and thus changed the course of my life. Without Reva (and Brené) I probably would not have had the courage and wisdom to ask James to take me back. I can't say a special thank you to every client, but here are a few more special shout-outs. Thank you Jenny and Julio (I always aim to "can to can"), Trixie and Danny (thank you for introducing "management" into my self-talk), Trudy, Charney (you make life "more better"), Marvin and Miriam, Annette (unicorn anyone?), Ines, Tanya (calmness is a superpower), Sue, Linda D., Andrea, Amy, Donna, Gayle, Mia, Bill and Alison (for giving me hope for relationships), Milan, Laura, Janice, Vicky and Clara, Julie L., Isa, Margaret, Barry, Karen, Trixie, Danielle, Fran, Daniela, Leah, Sue, Mel and Kelly, Sunita, Erin, Noah, Penny, Gayle, Michael, Natalie, Carol, Gabrielle, Linda R., Andrew, Karen and Barry, Odette, Lisa C., Lisa S., Alexi (love feeling the water off of a duck's back), Alex, Louise and Ric, Catherine, Natalie, and Maria.

Of course, thank you to everyone at Dundurn, including Kathryn Lane, Laura Boyle, Elena Radic, Kathryn Bassett, and Rachel Spence. I could not ask for a better publishing house. Kate Unrau, your edits made this book *so* much better! I miss you Jaclyn Hodsdon and Margaret Bryant — it was an honour to work with both of you on *Finding Your Fit*. Also, a big thank you to Jason Southerland and everyone at Dalyn Miller PR. Jason, I look forward to your peppy emails. You make PR fun.

And thank you, my readers. I am so excited and honoured to share in your search for your fittest future self!

About Kathleen

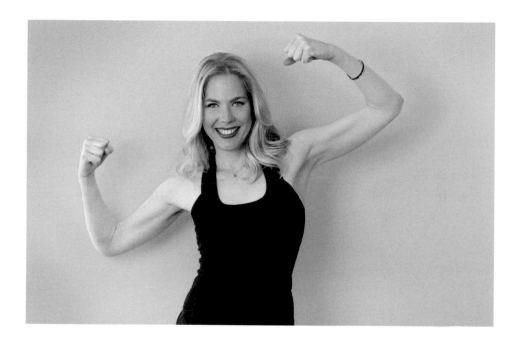

Kathleen Trotter is a fitness expert, media personality, personal trainer, writer, life coach, certified Pilates and ELDOA instructor, and overall health enthusiast. Her passion is motivating others to "find their fit." Kathleen does this through writing, regular TV and media appearances, working with clients (ranging from athletes of all ages to individuals living with Parkinson's disease and osteoporosis), and speaking engagements.

Kathleen holds an M.Sc. in Exercise Science from the University of Toronto and a nutrition diploma from the Canadian School of Natural Nutrition. She is a C.H.E.K. level 3 trainer, a level 2 Fascial

Stretch Therapist, a level 1 ELDOA practitioner, a certified pilates equipment specialist, and a level 2 life coach. In 2019, she will also become a certified Precision Nutrition coach.

Kathleen started her work as a fitness writer at *Chatelaine* in 2010. Shortly after, she started blogging for *the Huffington Post* and filming and writing for the *Globe and Mail.* Kathleen has published articles in magazines, such as *Canadian Running, Glow, Today's Parent, Healthy Directions, and Impact Magazine.*

She is regularly interviewed as a fitness expert for multiple news outlets including *Global* News and the *Toronto Star.* She also makes regular appearances on Breakfast Television Montreal, CTV News, Morning Live Hamilton, CBC, ABC News 7, and many others. Kathleen has been a guest on numerous radio shows and podcasts, and is a regular on Zoomer Radio's *The Tonic.*

Kathleen's new-found passion is motivational speaking. Her speaking engagements have included a series of motivational lectures hosted by the Toronto Public Library, guest lectures at the University of Toronto and Concordia University, Lunch and Learns at the University of Toronto, and corporate presentations, including her recent Cisco Women of Influence keynote talk.

Kathleen loves her job. Her mission is to inspire as many people as possible to adopt (in an intelligent way) a healthier lifestyle and to make healthier choices because they love themselves, not because they hate themselves. Kathleen does not believe in body shame. Kathleen does believe in goals and results. She does not believe in being "easy" on yourself or letting negative "brain propaganda" win. She does believe in self-compassion and holding yourself accountable. Kathleen does not believe in being active to create a whole new you. Kathleen does believe in being you, but working toward creating a you who has more healthy habits. She believes in learning and growing, passion, gratitude, and actively finding pockets of joy. Most important, Kathleen believes in actively creating the version of yourself that you want to be, and that the key to health success is finding YOUR fit — hence the name of her first book, *Finding Your Fit.*

Credits

• •

Photo Credits

AGNES KIESZ, PURE STUDIOS: cover, 235

TANIA CANNARELLA: 158, 159, 160, 188

CHARLES EBBS: 93, 124, 125, 126, 127, 132, 133, 136, 146, 147, 148, 149, 150, 151, 153, 154

Book Credits

PROJECT EDITOR: Elena Radic

DEVELOPMENTAL EDITOR: Kate Unrau

COPY EDITOR: Dawn Hunter

PROOFREADER: Emma Warnken-Johnson

COVER DESIGNER: Laura Boyle

INTERIOR DESIGNER: Courtney Horner

PUBLICIST: Elham Ali

Dundurn

PUBLISHER: J. Kirk Howard

VICE-PRESIDENT: Carl A. Brand

EDITORIAL DIRECTOR: Kathryn Lane

ARTISTIC DIRECTOR: Laura Boyle

PRODUCTION MANAGER: Rudi Garcia

DIRECTOR OF SALES AND MARKETING: Synora Van Drine

PUBLICITY MANAGER: Michelle Melski

MANAGER, ACCOUNTING AND TECHNICAL SERVICES: Livio Copetti

EDITORIAL: Allison Hirst, Dominic Farrell, Jenny McWha, Rachel Spence, Elena Radic, Melissa Kawaguchi

MARKETING AND PUBLICITY: Kendra Martin, Kathryn Bassett, Elham Ali, Tabassum Siddiqui, Heather McLeod

DESIGN AND PRODUCTION: Sophie Paas-Lang

By the Same Author

• •

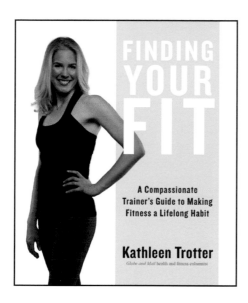

FINDING YOUR FIT: A COMPASSIONATE TRAINER'S GUIDE TO MAKING FITNESS A LIFELONG HABIT

Ten simple, practical ways to get moving, get healthy, and feel great.

Wanting to get on track and actually getting (and then staying) on track are two totally different things. The million-dollar question is: how do we find the inner motivation to go from thinking about a healthier lifestyle to actually adopting one? How do we get off the sofa and out the front door? *Finding Your Fit: A Compassionate Trainer's Guide to Making Fitness a Lifelong Habit* provides readers with practical tools that will allow them to connect the dots between wanting to make a health and fitness change, and actually making it.

dundurn.com    dundurnpress
@dundurnpress   dundurnpress
dundurnpress   info@dundurn.com

FIND US ON NETGALLEY & GOODREADS TOO!

DUNDURN